Healing Breast Cancer

A Spiritual and Medical Odyssey

Tara,
May God guide you in your journey. You are someone who has touched my life. Best Wishes to you always. You are in my prayers.
Always
Toni

Dorothy Elder

Healing Breast Cancer

A Spiritual and Medical Odyssey

This paperback edition published by

Doriel Publishing Company
Dorothy Elder
2557 South Dover, #75
Denver, Colorado 80227

Blessings
Dorothy Elder

ISBN 0-9631673-5-9

Table of Contents

Foreword

If serious illness comes into one's life, the first experience is probably shock. Then, if you are greatly blessed, there will be spiritual guidance that takes you through.

Dorothy Elder's book may be that guidance. Dorothy brings a profound gift to anyone who has had the devastating experience of any catastrophic illness. She writes clearly and beautifully from her own experience of breast cancer.

Dorothy guides you into the use of spiritual tools as part of a healing journey, even as she integrates them with medical processes. This integration may become yours.

The chapters on guidance from dreams and the process of inner voice dialogue (Active Imagination) are especially powerful and valuable. They are a guide into your own mystery of healing.

Rev. Marj Britt
Unity minister, Tustin, California

Preface

Some four and a half years ago, I was besieged by a very common disease—breast cancer. As a result I have been taught much about this popular disease that plagues so many women—young and old. Since I have been on my spiritual path for over thirty years I did not expect such a challenge but since my Purpose is to write and publish spiritual books for seekers of Truth, perhaps I had this challenge to teach me what I needed to heal in my own life and to learn firsthand what thousands of women are going through. I have deep empathy and compassion for each one. In order to really understand challenges of others, we may have the same one.

At the beginning I was inspired to keep a Journal describing the entire procedure and my learning. After my healing I brought it together in a book entitled, *Healing Breast Cancer: A Spiritual and Medical Odyssey.* It was a very personal account, of course, but I also gave my experience in hopes that other women challenged with the same problem would gain strength and direction. It was quite lengthy and very personal. I submitted it to publishers but it was turned down. After three years I was guided to write a shorter, more universal version. Thus the birth of this book. I refer often to personal responses to the Journey but my main theme is "You can be healed."

Introduction

A Personal Account

And God said to me, "My Grace is sufficient
for you for power is perfected
in weakness."
2 Corinthians 12:9

The beginning of this introduction was written early in my challenge with breast cancer. A complete Journal of each day's experiences described ups and downs. I wanted to write a book when I was healed about the experience and the various ups and downs I faced. I wrote in my Journal:

> *Here I am in the middle of a great challenge. I will not say it is my greatest challenge, but a challenge that requires a lifting of consciousness of my Divinity, or I will not be healed. For it is beholden upon me to write this account in order to help other women to whom this challenge may come. There is a healing of the big "C" waiting for those who find their Journey focused on spiritual and medical routes to healing.*

This book came from that challenge. The successful medical practice, the deep alliance with a spiritual healer, and the use of the alternative healing acupuncture has brought the reward of complete healing. I am into my fifth year of freedom from that challenge. The following is offered as a witness to the very human/spiritual life I have lived. It is not so different from the lives of many women who have not had this devastating disease strike. But for many, I hope, it will offer healing guidance.

This autobiography was written early in my challenge and later.

I am 85 years old. I have lived a comparatively healthy life, according to physical standards. I have had many challenges—psychologically, physically, emotionally, religiously, and indeed in relationships. The latter seems to be the area in which I have had the most challenges and through which God has expanded my consciousness of who I am.

A brief résumé of my life seems in order.

I was born into a family of four brothers on a farm in Oklahoma. We moved to a farm in New Mexico when I was seven. The Depression was in full swing during my teen years. I attended college for two years and married a schoolteacher who was deeply religious. We had three children: two girls and a boy. My husband eventually quit teaching and went into the car dealership business with his father and brother in Texas. There we raised our children.

After twenty years of trying to find peace and happiness in that marriage, I obtained a Bachelor's degree and subsequently a divorce. After teaching school two years, I obtained a Master's degree in counseling adolescents, moved to Colorado, counseled in high school for sixteen years, retired, and started writing books at age 62. Years later, when the books were published and selling very well, I knew I was fulfilling my purpose, finally.

At age 50, my life took a complete turnaround. All of my life I had sought a relationship with God. I did not grow up in a religious home. I married a man whose religious beliefs did not satisfy my longing. I studied psychology to find answers but realized it lacked what I needed for my peace. Then I discovered Carl Jung's teachings—a combination of psychology and spirituality—and found many answers to my quest. But I was still relying on outer authority to teach me.

And then I had the challenge of challenges. In late 1966, I received word that my son had been killed in Vietnam.

He had chosen to enlist in late 1965, was not drafted. He had been in Vietnam as a "foot soldier" for five months when he was shot while on patrol. My heart was broken, but a precognitive dream had prepared me more than I realized at the time. That opening, through the dream really, led me to my spiritual seeking. He left a wife, who was pregnant. It was her love and caring, as well as her sharing their son later with me, that helped assuage the sorrow. But there was still a vacancy and I recognized it as a spiritual one.

As I have said, challenges in relationships seem to be my Path this time around. These challenges have, of course, forced me to seek a higher Path and to find my Christ, my life, my purpose. It is my Odyssey.

I started seeking answers to Why? Why? Why? How do I find peace again? What do I need in my life to bring me to a closer walk with God? Where is surcease from pain to be found? Where do I look? I have a successful career, health, many friends, family, etc. But it is not enough. I am hurting and all of this success helps, but it does not heal the deep grief over the loss of my son.

The answers did not come immediately. I was guided to my search. I will not go into all details. I know now that God was guiding me, was leading me, was assuring me that the answers lay in fulfilling my spiritual quest. And that would come. So books, teachers, classes, groups, inspiration dropped into my life, into my experience, into my thoughts, into my heart. I learned that a broader perspective on my spiritual Odyssey was required. I found *that* in the commonalities of the religions of the ages, the religions of the world.

As I searched, I was led to a metaphysical church. I found that those teachings were actually what my inner Self was revealing to me. I was delighted. I had attended many other churches looking for confirmation of what seemed truth to me, but had not found it. Here in the metaphysical I was rewarded.

The first step for me was control of my thoughts through affirmation of the good and denial of the not-so-good. I studied at the central school, learned about metaphorical interpretation of the Bible, and grew in spiritual awareness. This was a good start. Turning within in meditation was touched on, but prayer was emphasized. Meditation came later for me.

Much later I realized that I was stepping on the mystic path as my consciousness expanded to Oneness with All there is. This move to centeredness on the Inner Spirit became my Guide.

Little by little, my grieving was assuaged over my son's death. I was still resentful of our government and its involvement in a useless Vietnam War. Of course, I was not always Centered—much more meditation was needed. I learned that the Spirit within, God in all, is soul. I came to realize that this was a common teaching of all religions under various names. I was then drawn to that Spirit within, consciously, through my study and my spiritual practice of meditation.

I overcame lots of skepticism. My education, my childhood's lack of religious teaching, my experience with my husband and his fundamentalist belief had blocked my inner voice. I then traveled to learn about people of the world and their religions. I finished my counseling career as a high school counselor, I found Jungian dream interpretation, which cleared me of many shadows, and I retired. By this time I was deeply immersed in my spiritual Journey. It was primary in my life. Six months before retirement, I was given a commission from Holy Spirit to write my first book, *Revelation for a New Age*, based on the book of Revelation in the New Testament of the Bible. And a whole new life opened for me. I became a successful writer and publisher.

When I was given the gift of creativity to write that interpretation, my consciousness expanded exponentially, and I began studying the Bible more deeply. I had been writing poetry for several years and accepted that as a gift from God for my own spiritual Path. I had been meditating deeply, I listened to my Inner Voice, and let it come forth in words revealing deep spiritual truth. That led me to letting go of my intellect and depending on intuitive knowing, and thus I was able to write that interpretation of the Book of Revelation. Success in getting it published quickly added to my reassurance that I was here to share metaphorical interpretations of the Bible with seekers. Thus, I have written fourteen books, seven of which have been published. My deep study, my own spiritual awakening, the teaching of my teachers through books, classes and especially inspiration led me on.

My first three books were published by a national publisher. They were popular. Later I self-published an additional four books.

I was healthy, had many spiritual friends, and was fulfilled with my creative endeavors. I had experience of bliss from the flowing of my Divine Energy. I thought I was nearly enlightened. Boy, what ego! No, no. I had "many miles to cover" before I would arrive.

And then I discovered a small growth on my breast. Being a good metaphysical student and somewhat a mystic, I decided to ignore it. I prayed, I treated, I declared that it would disappear. It was no-thing. It was an illusion. It was not real. It would fade away. I did not want to face what so many women were facing—a disease on my breast. My ego was having a field day! After all, I told myself, I was deep into meditation, into my spiritual Journey. My books were selling well. I was writing from my intuition, from my Inner Consciousness—and my readers were finding answers for their spiritual journey. So I couldn't have a glitch in my Path. Could I? Ego, move over.

It grew slowly. I ignored. No pain. No need to seek a doctor, I thought. I told myself I did not need a mammogram. I thought the medical world was building up this fear of cancer to prove they were right. Besides, they did not really know how to heal breast cancer. Finally, after about a year of playing this game, the lump was larger, and I went for an examination.

My medical Odyssey is described in Chapter III.

Years before this challenge my two daughters had married and were living in other states. Carolyn, the youngest, had two children and was busy with work and family responsibilities. Sue, likewise, was married and had a son. I had visited each frequently. They had also visited me. I was on my spiritual Path and had written and published two books. And then I had a deep challenge. Both of my daughters separated from me for various reasons. I mention this here because healing those separations became a large part of my Path to healing.

As I have studied those mystics who gave up all for their spiritual journey to Allness, I have realized that having a deep spiritual commitment <u>may</u> bring separation from family, friends, other relationships. This is difficult to accept when one has carried doubts about one's own ability to be successful in relationships. Guilt and fear accrue. But one on the spiritual Path will finally realize that centeredness on one's own spiritual journey may bring challenges, separations but a longing for relationships. These are filled with the Divine Being, Love, which is needed in order to follow one's spiritual purpose. New relationships develop based on spiritual love. It took me years to accept this as the healing of the separation from my daughters. Many times these broken relationships are restored as one expands consciousness of the God of Being. But sometimes the separation needs to be accepted, blessed, and released with love.

After several years of silence from my daughters and my experiencing my mother complex of grieving, trying to make amends, forgiving myself and them, I gave up. I thought that they had to find themselves, find their own path without interference from me. They needed to live their own lives separate from me. I was deeply grieved, unconsciously if not consciously. The separation did not heal. And I was now facing the need to try again.

As I began recognizing the seriousness of the lump on my breast, I began considering where I may have blocked love from my heart chakra, which could have caused the results in my breast. This came from my years of studying Jungian psychology and spirituality as well as many examples that I had observed. I believed that what we think and feel, or don't think and feel, can cause interference with the flow of that Divine Energy called kundalini, chi, ki, Holy Spirit, which produces and renews health. I then realized that I needed to contact my daughters to unblock the flow of love. (See Chapter II for an account of that healing.)

Now this is not a unique story about breast cancer for I have learned how many other women have gone through this challenge and have gained a deeper appreciation for love, faith, and a new direction for their life and have been healed. The healings are often covered up by the accounts of the deaths from this disease, but there are many healings and women are telling their story in order to help other women find their own healing. In the long run, each of us, although advised by our doctors as to the course of treatment for healing, look for guidance to help in the healing process, often from our own spiritual inner center. Thus it was for me.

Perhaps the method that brought success to my healing will bring inspiration to other women who do not know where to turn to find peace and lose much fear that society, the medical world, and other women's experiences impose on them. My purpose is to tell my story, hoping it will inspire others to find their own personal path to healing. I pray that healing of body, mind, feelings with spirit will result.

I shall make some of my account brief. Other parts of it will be longer and deeper for what I am to reveal is based on my philosophy and on scripture. "My Grace is sufficient for you, for power is perfected in weakness."[1] That is a deep Truth.

There were five commitments I practiced to be healed. They are: (1) Healing relationships with loved ones, (2) Having traditional medical therapy, (3) Following teachings by a spiritual teacher, (4) Long and deep meditation, and (5) Alternative healing through acupuncture. For me, these all were necessary. As a result, I have found greater peace emotionally, physically, mentally, and spiritually. There are great blessings that can come from one's challenges!

My hope is that women who may be going through this deep, dark cavern of breast cancer may be able to relate to some of my experiences and thus find answers to their journey through this great challenge. I found the real healer to be that Inner Counselor, Comforter, Spirit of Truth as Jesus named the Holy Spirit. Medical, spiritual and alternative healing supported my healing.

Let us go now to those chapters that describe my Odyssey.

CHAPTER I

Accepting My Need For Healing

As I have followed the accounts of other women who deal with this challenge, I am impressed with how similar our stories are. Some of us are aware of a lump in the breast for some time but ignore it. In some healing philosophy it is taught one should ignore and go through positive healing practices each day. And it works for many. But for the rest of us, honesty about needing a mammogram may save our lives. On the other hand, fear will continue unless our faith keeps us aware of a possible healing.

I was aware of the lump in my breast for a long time. It was small and did not get larger and there was no pain. I had a dream about losing my way on my spiritual Journey and another dream of separation from my son and daughters. The later dream made me realize that I was not free of the pain of those separations, which could be the cause of the lump on my breast. I needed to work on that separation of my two daughters as well as seek medical evaluation. Remember, I was a very independent woman, unmarried, a retired high school counselor, a serious Seeker for Truth and a successful author of spiritual books. I had ego. I thought, "This could not be serious. I am living a spiritual life and am protected by the love of God." Yes indeed! But I needed reassurance. I needed to face the truth.

Other women may put off the initial examination for other reasons. Fear, depression, no support from close relationships, no time to go to the doctor, no insurance and an overwhelming need to pretend that all is well. When one is so busy caring for children, husband, perhaps aged parents, there is no time for one's own mental and physical health. That is a mistake. One is playing an end game. The quicker one starts on treatment the better. Of course, some women are not aware of a lump. Perhaps a mammogram should be routine for many.

I knew nothing about breast lump examination. I had never had one. So I was very leery of going to any doctor. I finally went to a clinic and had a mammogram. The lump was pictured and a biopsy was recommended. I was reluctant but finally agreed. One warning—be sure you find the right doctor. Sometimes the one that is recommended does not fit one's personality and physical needs. Find one that is right for you!

I was referred to a surgeon, a specialist in breast cancer, a woman. She did a biopsy, which revealed the cancer cells. This doctor was just right for me. She treated me with respect for my wishes and was really interested in my healing. She also respected my independent questions and decisions.

I wrote in my original manuscript as I went through the healing:

> *I must also say again that I found that I had to weigh the choices that I made about this healing. One must not give up her own authority. Decisions need to be made. The seeker for healing must not allow another person to make all the decisions without respect for the patient. One who practices prayer and meditation has the advantage of being able to quiet thoughts, go within and listen for guidance. Seek advice from other doctors or seek advice from another one who has gone through the same experience.*

The result of learning that the lump was cancerous brought forth a midnight message to allay my fear. Since spirituality had played such an important part in my life for 30 years, I wondered:

> *I am at the crossroads of my life. I am being tested. Do I follow science or do I follow spirituality? They seem to be divided at this point. Do I look for medical healing or do I look to spiritual healing, God-healing? This is a vital decision in my life. Or are medical and spiritual healings both the same? Do they come from the same source?*

After a deep meditation and prayer I let go and let God guide me. Fear had entered in but I knew I was being taken care of. So I chose all three—prayer, spiritual healing and medical healing. That was a most important decision. They worked in tandem for me. I knew that this challenge would bring me to opening myself up to God-healing as well as medical healing, which is the same. I was at peace.

From my experience I would strongly suggest that women faced with this challenge find a spiritual practitioner who gives healing prayers through meditation and turn to them with full confidence in the healing result of faith in God. There are many available now. Those attached and trained in a New Thought teaching may be your choice. Let Spirit and the medical healing relate, be at One. Fear is not in the cancer. When we surrender human identity to the I AM we have taken a major step. Philippians 4:13: "I can do all things in him who strengthens me."[2]

Do not forget—fear will enter in now and then. But let go and turn to the peace that your Spirit can bring. Let God be God.

I had an MRI and then made an appointment with an oncologist who was recommended by the surgeon. He and I became close friends as well as being my teacher. I was guided to the right doctors!

Chapter II

Healing Physical and Emotional Pain

I had taken care of the medical/physical requirements to start healing breast cancer. I had followed the scientific way. But because I believe that a physical challenge is also an emotional and spiritual challenge, I went deeply into my unconscious to recognize what needed healing there. And so I became quiet and listened through Active Imagination.

Active Imagination is a term Carl Jung used to solve problems and to gain Inner Inspiration for one's life. I became quiet as I rested and realized that the healing of an emotional separation was needed. And I was separated from my two daughters through various misunderstandings over the years.

Why do so many women have devastating diseases of breast cancer? Well, there can be many reasons but as I researched what emotional loss, a blockage of love from the heart chakra might affect the breast, I accepted that it might be that love Energy was blocked in that particular area of the body. As I accepted this as a possible reason for my breast cancer I knew my need to clear up the separation from each daughter. It took humility and spiritual support to proceed.

I had a blockage. I thought that maybe I should give up and let go of any attachment to them. But my Inner Self revealed that my unconscious grief would not go away by accepting the separation without trying to reach them. I was guided to turn to further spiritual Guidance to deal with the problem. I needed to forgive myself and them. I realized that my love feelings were still there and were blocked in expression.

I asked my Inner Self how I could release my love for them completely. The answer—

Journal:

> *Change your thinking. Free your love to be active. Turn within and listen for Guidance. Forgive and let love flow.* *

Then I went forth with the conviction that through love I would reach out again to each and pray for God's Guidance. I accepted that I might not be successful in renewing our relationships but it was God's will that I try, with great humility and strength. I was strengthened by love even if the relationships did not become closer. Suffering can open our hearts to taking action to heal.

Dr. Dean Ornish has published a book, *Love and Survival, the Scientific Basis for the Healing Power of Intimacy.* He stresses many times how lack of love given or received can cause cancer, especially breast cancer, to develop. He writes of several research projects that prove the need to forgive another and let love flow. He writes that many times a lack of closeness with parents or other important people brings on the challenge. He strongly recommends group involvement of cancer patients or those who have been healed as a means of opening up and expressing love for each other and to expand closer personal relationships that need healing.

Caroline Myss, in her book, *Anatomy of the Spirit*, wrote that healing begins with the repair of emotional injuries. The need to love ourselves and to have no separation in loving others is a requirement for a spiritual Journey. And healing of

---

*Quotes from my Journal are in italics.

many diseases comes through acts of forgiveness. She suggests that our personal, emotional challenges are extensions of a Divine plan, which intent is our conscious evolution. Oh boy! Is that the Truth for me! Illness, she wrote, is often a catalyst for spiritual transformation.

Bernie S. Siegel, M.D., wrote in his book, *Love, Medicine & Miracles*: To some extent cancer is not a primary disease. It is partly a reaction to a set of circumstances that weaken the body's defenses. Healing must address the patient's entire life.

Brugh Joy, M.D., in his book, *Joy's Way*, wrote: Most cancer patients have experienced emotional upsets within two years before the onset of the disease. To heal, major changes in their lives were sought. He suggests that psychological areas must be cleared that allow the disease to manifest in the body. He writes a great deal on the Energy of the chakra system. The Energy of the heart chakra feeds love into the body, mind, and feelings, which affect the breast. If it is blocked then disease may occur.

Back to my dilemma. I realized that expansion of my consciousness had occurred as I gave forgiveness to my daughters and their chosen separation. I could feel deeper compassion for others who were wounded. I had become closer in consciousness with the Christ. But I still had work to do for my own health and spiritual expansion as well as theirs. These ideas came to me to heal the separation.

Journal:

Feel love each time I thought of each daughter.
Live in the NOW. Let go of the past and no concern about the future.
Know that God's Will is my fulfillment.
Be positive in thought and feeling about them.
Love my Self and express that love freely to others.
Let go of small self-will and depend on God of the Universe.
Free each to be who they chose to be.

I started writing letters to my older daughter Sue, who I had not heard from for ten years, asking for forgiveness and explaining my serious challenge of breast cancer. She lived in the Chicago area with her husband, who was born in East India. Her son was grown and I had no idea where he was. She is a beautiful, intelligent woman who has chosen her own life style. She had been a great blessing to me and her father.

As I continued to send letters asking to hear from her, I received only silence. The letters were delivered—not a one was returned—so I knew she received them. But silence was her response.

I realized that expansion of my love chakra was necessary for my healing. My Inner Guidance shouted: "Wait! Wait! Wait!"

I finally freed Sue at Christmas as I continued my medical and spiritual healing. Since she had not responded I did not want to impose on her. I remembered the joy I had had as her mother and I hoped she realized my love and would forgive me in the future. An Inner Message came to me—

Journal:

Let go of pursuing this relationship. Let go of expectation of a reply from her now. Continue loving her. Your healing will be enhanced as you turn within and let the Holy Spirit speak to you and to her. Free Sue in love.

I realized:

She will always be in my heart for she has been a great blessing to me. Her soul's Journey is her important task all of her life.

I am reminded that at Christmas, broken relationships take on a darker hue. Thus I have had the dream and soul searching about Sue. I release all to God's Will. I rest in that Will. I shall send her a card occasionally and send her love and joy in my meditation, a healing time.

I am learning another lesson, which I need. The past is gone. NOW is and I AM. The present is all I have. God is my life and I have followed Her guidance. I had another lesson to learn—let go of all relationships to Her guidance. She is caring for Sue and for me. She, the Mother God, is bringing to me an opportunity to love unconditionally and without attachment. All is well. I have freed Sue. If the Spirit brings us together in the future, I shall rejoice, but I know we are together spiritually now. We are One—her Christ and mine.

I have listened to a Goldsmith tape on love loaned to me. I began to wonder: Was I separated from God when I decided to put my daughters out of my thought and feelings some years ago? Yes. I (my small self) took over. My small self was hurt. I wanted to protect it. My Self was blocked, my Self which is Love. My love ceased to flow to them and I had this blockage, this knot, over my heart. This is a sign of the love that was clamoring for attention. Love heals, nothing else. I am healed because love is the center of my choices. I am love. When I block love, I block that Holy Spirit which is All. My Body is teaching me. My body is Holy. It has caught my attention and I have returned to the Path of Love.

Carolyn, my other daughter, is younger than Sue by 19 months. She is also intelligent and beautiful. She has been more independent of my influence than Sue. After she started to college at some distance from our home, she matured quickly. Her father and grandfather had great influence over her choices. But we still had a mother and daughter relationship for many years, which was deep at times.

She married and divorced, had two children, was a successful businesswoman. We had drifted apart several times during the years but were friends and loved each other dearly.

In the Fall of my discovery, I received a card from her on my birthday. She wrote that she loved me and thanked me for giving her life. I was so grateful to hear from her.

Journal:

> *It was her God-Self that contacted me. She, like most of us, has great love but because of fear, we may not express it. That is true of me also at times. I accept her as she is—human and divine—and love and pray for her.*

I answered her card by thanking her for being my daughter and told her of my challenge and asked her forgiveness and freed her to her chosen path. My challenge opened up a whole new loving conversation. She replied with a wonderful loving letter and said she would call me as soon as she got settled in Mexico for the winter. And she did and we had months of close loving contact. She had gone through the challenge of a possible breast cancer examination but the growth was benign. She understood my challenge. We had several telephone conversations before she left her summer home to go to Mexico.

Carolyn was not in contact with Sue either. Contact with Carolyn helped me get through the weeks and months of treatment. It was a great gift of love that Carolyn and I talked about frequently. I called her on her birthday and thanked her for her understanding and loving attention.

Carolyn was separated from her husband although they remained friends. She had challenges in relationships sometimes as we all do. Her personality was so deeply loving that sometimes she often made choices that "backfired". A human fallacy!! Our many phone conversations allowed her to share with me and I with her, of course.

As time went by she called to check my progress and I felt her loving concern. She was enjoying new friends in Mexico, had started a job selling real estate. Her joyful response when I spoke of my healing lifted me up. She understood the decisions that I had to make and helped me.

When in March of 1998 I had a lumpectomy after a series of chemotherapy treatments, Carolyn expressed her love for me in spirit and she was so glad that I was healed.

Just before Christmas, nine months after my healing, she arrived for an extended visit. We celebrated Christmas at a special hotel in Colorado Springs. It was so wonderful to have a daughter with me. But then she asked me a question about her daughter, who was married and had a baby. Her daughter had been estranged from her mother for several years. I answered it honestly and she went into a deep depression. Then she decided to return to her home in Mexico early as she was so upset with me. Our relationship became silent again. I was sorry she was so deeply affected by what she called lack of devotion to her as my daughter. My need was to be honest with her as I answered her question.

I have wondered if I should have been less direct with my answer. My perception of my granddaughter's hurt was one of deep sympathy but perhaps I should have softened my reply to Carolyn's question. One's perception of honesty may change as the feelings of the people involved need to be considered. My answer could have been less vigorous with more feeling of sympathy for how it would affect my daughter. I answered her question but I should have said, "Why don't you ask her. I am a third party." Difficulties between two parties can only be settled between them.

I was unable to contact her for I did not know her address and she remained silent.

I went through grief, of course, as I was grieved by the separation. My mother attachment caused me emotional pain. But the Presence of God brought me through to a like decision as I had accepted about Sue's silence. Carolyn had her own physical and spiritual mission to fulfill. If it did not include any of her original family, I had to accept that. I released her to her

Good. I continue to send love and compassion to her and bless her.

Many parents of grown children are having these challenges with them and sometimes at a very young age. When one or other party decides to break the connection only love and prayer and forgiveness can bring a healing. To find a path back to a loving, forgiving relationship is important but if it fails then only prayer and release through understanding can bring peace.

These experiences with my daughters brought home to me that one's Purpose as a woman may not be in finding one's emotional food through mother/child relationships but through Holy Spirit guidance to fulfill one's spiritual Purpose. A broken relationship may not include continued motherhood to daughters and sons. Sometimes we must free them to find their own Purpose. My love and divine wishes go with each daughter. They are Free, Free, Free. And so am I!

I have included this account for it is definitely a part of my healing of breast cancer as well as a step forward emotionally, physically, and mentally for them and me. I practice love much more deeply and feed my mother breasts with that Divine Energy. I go forth to share with others my lesson as well as my healing. Thus I pray that facing my challenge, physically, emotionally, and spiritually, may help many others. Love, compassion, understanding and prayer strengthen one.

Here I am, four years after my healing of breast cancer, and I have accepted that I had not been a perfect mother and had failed my children in many ways as they grew up. We as mothers are such novices. We learn by doing and make mistakes. When I began to focus on my education and teachings to free myself from an unhappy marriage, they were affected. Now my Purpose in writing and publishing books has helped many of my readers. It is a big price to pay but who knows, perhaps this was my spiritual destiny. They are blessed on their Way!

I turned to my spiritual teacher, Elizabeth.

Journal:

I called Elizabeth. She gave me another teaching on All is Spirit. I told her I thought she was very patient with me as she has taught me the same lesson over and over, and I did not seem to get it. She laughed. To realize the truth of the Infinite Way, Goldsmith's teaching, is one thing. To practice it in thought, word and deed is another. She said, "You have reached that knowing in personal security and supply. All that is left is to have the same knowing for health. Go for it."

She is correct. Negative emotions are also an interference to health of body and mind. Through love, those are and will be cleared of any blockage to health.

I have realized that my daughters and I are not really separated for in the Spirit we are all One. Our belief in separation changes when we accept the Reality that we are all One spiritually. Our belief of separation is based more on our differences physically, emotionally and mentally. But the truth is that our spiritual perception is beyond belief in separation. Jesus taught: "The Father and I are One." (John 10:30) And Galatians 3:28 reads: "There is no longer Jew or Greek, there is no longer slave or free, there is no longer male and female; for all of you are One in Christ Jesus."

Oneness is the mystic realm to which we all aspire spiritually. Oneness is our Truth. We are not separate. We are One spiritually.

As we pursue our Path to conscious awareness that there are no failures, only lessons on our way to full consciousness of our Oneness. I have learned much spiritually from this lesson.

Oneness is our Truth.

CHAPTER III

The Medical Healing

Hearing the final results—that there were cancer cells in the tumor in my breast—shook me up. I guess I had played the game well—it is malignant! My surgeon was very direct. She recommended an oncologist whom she respected highly and asked me to make an appointment. She understood my shock and was gentle.

About one o'clock the next morning as fear arose, I affirmed, "I see and feel God all around and through me. I let go of any fear. I let go of clinging to thoughts of the scientist. This body is God's body, not mine as a human. It is my choice to trust God. I let God be God."

That took away my fear. I declared, "I will be healed. The growth is an illusion, not truth." This was pure Spiritual healing.

As I finished these affirmations I knew that this challenge had large opportunities as I went through the healing. Opportunities for my spiritual expansion and opportunities for those who would read the book that I would write about the experience.

In spite of this spiritual cleansing, I found fear still entering my thoughts and feelings. The possibility that I might die due to this disease surfaced. I had no fear of death but I realized there were mundane matters to be taken care of. So I began the process of writing a new will.

I was pretty ignorant about cancer therapy and I found a book that was written by a cancer specialist. *Dr. Susan Love's Breast Book*, was written by Susan M. Love, M.D., with Karen Lindsey. It filled in some answers that I didn't have time to ask the surgeon or oncologist.

One needs to be a part of some of the decisions made by the doctor. He asked me to be in a research project but because I do not approve of those research projects when one group is given treatment that is expected to heal and the other group may not receive the treatment, I turned it down. He accepted my decision graciously.

As I have written, I liked the oncologist immediately. He was a man with a large cancer healing practice and at the head of a group of cancer specialists. He was in total cooperation with the surgeon's suggestion that I have chemo before the operation. He understood that to reduce the size of the tumor was important. Four chemo treatments were suggested.

As we chatted I told him I was keeping a Journal and planned to write a book on my challenge. He said he wanted to read it and he did read the original manuscript and later wrote a recommendation for publishers that I submitted the manuscript to.

It had been five weeks since my first examination by a doctor. Now I was going to plan a schedule for treatment. I wondered why it took so long or was that really a short wait. I learned that there are so many women seeking this treatment that sometimes it takes a while to get started. I was certainly ignorant of the procedure. However, I realized that cooperation with the medical world was very important. When I chose my oncologist I trusted him to be as interested in my healing as I was.

The oncologist insisted on a complete physical examination—an EKG, a bone scan, an ultra-sound of my gall bladder and other organs. It was tiring but I came through with flying colors.

As one goes into treatment it is well to not read about the failures of different cancer treatments. Also negative news on TV, radio and the press should be bypassed. These planted in one's mind can affect the healing process. Fear may block healing Energy in body, thought and feeling. Faith and quieting all fear-filled thoughts are necessary. Also, talking about the challenge to friends and relatives should be bypassed. Their fear-filled thoughts and/or spoken words may affect the patient's healing.

As I waited for my first chemo treatment, which I was totally ignorant about, I had a dream. I dreamed about a man named Cosmo who entered into a group conversation with deep knowledge. I was totally at ease with him. I interpreted the dream (see Chapter VII, Dream Time Related to Healing) as seeing Cosmo as short for Cosmos, which symbolizes order and harmony. I accepted that order and harmony would accompany me through this challenge and it did.

A young nurse introduced me to the chemotherapy procedure and its possible outcome. She laid a negative scene. I told her that I did not expect the negative result or procedure as she had outlined. Later she gave me a printout by the oncologist that presented a positive introduction to chemotherapy.

After this meeting, a positive spiritual teaching came through: "I AM in the medicine. I AM in the scientist that developed the healing method. I AM that chemo. I AM THE HEALING. Nothing is separate from Me."

A patient can block the healing method by various psychological and mental blocks, it is believed. Fear, lack of belief in the healing method, and various other reasons to disbelieve may occur. For my philosophy I saw no separation between the medical and spiritual healing in combination. Those who are healed will recognize this and go into the world to teach and live it. I heard, "I AM ALL." Beautiful! I knew Truth had been given to me.

In a sense this experience had been a crucifixion for me. A crucifixion of many mental, emotional and physical rules that I seemed to live by. I was inspired: "Through this crucifixion I shall be resurrected and ascend into higher, more complete Oneness of consciousness. I will teach others through the book I shall write and those who come to me."

On November 11, I had my first chemo. I had started this healing procedure on September 11, 1997. Just a warning—be patient, your healing treatment will come. Be ready!

A friend was to drive me to the doctor's office for the first treatment and later spend the night with me. This was a cautious procedure that I did not need but other patients may accept the kind offering of dear friends to help out. My treatments did not affect me negatively so I could care for myself.

As I entered the office I was asked to sign a consent form, which removed all responsibility from the doctor for a long list of potential problems. He was protected. Then to the treatment room.

The treatment was painless and lasted ninety minutes. I was given some pills to take home in case of nausea.

Journal:

First night and after first chemo: I was restless and awoke several times. Once I felt nauseous. I turned within. I "saw" a flash of a man surrounded by Light. Knew it was my Guide, perhaps Jesus Christ. I became quiet, felt the beautiful silence. Difficult to describe. It was Wholeness, Allness, Stillness, Fullness. No words can describe it. I slept. No nausea. I am healed. The Energy has washed me clean.

Each doctor has his/her own procedure for the chemo treatment. I was comfortable with the procedure my oncologist had arranged. After each chemo treatment I had to return to the laboratory for three days to have my blood count checked for white blood cells. I was given a shot of Neupogen at each examination if I needed it. Otherwise I did not have an extreme negative experience except perhaps a day or two of dis-ease. Constipation was a continual problem. Pills provided by the doctor eased that at times.

At one point I had a deep ache in the lump. It became more and more painful. It was extremely painful for a short time and then the pain receded. Was I having a healing by the Spirit within? I wondered. The experience was as though some energy was pressing from within as well as from without.

There were negative times resulting from the chemo. I lost all of my hair, so bought a wig. Got many compliments from friends who thought it was my natural hair. Also, my depth of spiritual awareness increased and my spiritual counselor's teaching and meditation was so healing and quieted my concerns.

Chemo treatment is a strange experience. Each has her own experience. I had four treatments with three weeks between each one. And the after-effects were not always the same.

There are spiritual healers who have been successful in healing breast cancer in a client. Since I did not have that experience I cannot speak with authority but I believe it can happen. I needed medical as well as spiritual and energy healing. If the woman is healed without her changing the direction of her life, which may lack love received or given, she may be afflicted again. Or perhaps not. The reason for breast cancer is still not agreed upon. The spiritual healer can bring Light to the Seeker but the Seeker has the responsibility of changing his/her own consciousness by turning to that Holy Spirit and praying and meditating often. Also study of spiritual healing can be helpful.

I went through periods of great peace and joy as I knew I was healing. Then I would drop down where I was not at peace. The chemicals inserted in my body always caused a period of unrest. I was uplifted by the cheerfulness of many of the patients being treated in the same room. Others were of course downcast. It is a personal individual journey.

As I met with my oncologist now and then I was uplifted by his positive approach. I told him I was considering having acupuncture treatments as supplemental healing. He agreed it would be fine and many times asked me how it was going. As the lump became smaller due to the chemo treatments, he suggested March 4 as the date for the surgery. It was set up by my surgeon.

Now I should like to explain acupuncture treatment and how it helped in my healing.

Acupuncture

I was two months into my healing program when I decided to have acupuncture treatments as well as the chemo and surgery. I talked to my oncologist about my choice and he was fully supportive.

I had experienced healing by acupuncture some years previous. I had arthritis and chose to seek a chiropractor who used acupuncture to heal. I had gone to a traditional medical doctor who had diagnosed my aches, pains and swelling as arthritis. He wanted to start me on drugs to relieve my pain. I declined and found the chiropractor through a friend's recommendation. He treated me for some time and the pain and swelling left my body. That convinced me that acupuncture works. I have no arthritis now, years later. Of course, I was deep into spirituality at the same time.

Attraction to acupuncture was supported by my own spiritual investigation and study of the Divine Energy, life energy, which flows through our body. It is called *kundalini, chi, ki* by Eastern religionists. I learned that China has used this Energy for thousands of years to heal and it is still a most popular form of healing there along with other Eastern healing choices. It is also becoming well known and used in the West. Because this Energy activity in the body had become such truth for me in my study of Hinduism and Buddhism as well as having my own awakening of that spiritual Energy within my body and consciousness, I knew that it was the treatment I needed. Therefore as I faced this major physical, emotional and mental challenge, I knew it would enhance the healing of breast cancer.

My chiropractor had retired and I found another through the recommendation of a friend. Soon after I mentioned my plan to my oncologist I made an appointment.

Before I tell about the healing treatment I want to explain acupuncture as it is taught by the chiropractor/acupuncturist to whom I went.

For thousands of years the Chinese doctors have used acupuncture to heal physical illness. Acupressure, Tai Chi and other Chinese practices with healing energy were used. The body has electrical currents, which can be blocked and cause pain, illness and loss of mobility. When the body is healthy the energy is flowing freely. Health prevails. This energy is often referred to as life force, chi. In the Hindu teaching it is called kundalini. In Western teaching it is referred to as Divine Energy, Holy Spirit, also life energy.

When the body is balanced, is healthy, it is a sign that the energy is flowing freely. Tension in thoughts, emotions and physical injury can cause a blockage of the flow. Then pain and sickness may result. Opening the channels by insertion of needles in special points in the body releases the life flow. The acupuncturist has extensive training in the location of the points in the body.

To open the flow, the doctor may also use ultrasound at a low frequency. Chi Gong energy can also be applied from a vibrating instrument. This awakens the energy at a particular body location. Laser is also used in appropriate locations.

Healing, according to my doctor, is successful for ulcers, acne, migraine headaches, and any relief of pain. Also spinal adjustment often accompanies the acupuncture treatment.

My experience of no pain from the insertion of the needles just below the surface of the skin was one reason I believed in it. For some patients there may be a little discomfort but for most seekers, the treatment causes no pain and seems to work. However, in my opinion, the reason for the body reacting in pain and sickness may be caused by mental, emotional and spiritual imbalance. Those need attention also. My acupuncturist never mentioned the possible reason for the illness. He did ask if I was under any emotional or mental pressure.

His kindness and deep interest in my healing was great. He often told me that he learned so much from each of his patients, which improved his knowledge and practice. (See the tape by Kevin Woodard.)

My desire was for greater free flow of the Divine Energy throughout my body to help it balance the chemo treatments as well as to heal. Chi Gong, energy vibration, was placed on the lump area at times and on the solar plexus and the second chakra center (the sex chakra).

My attitude in being relaxed and accepting the healing in the treatment was an important part of the experience. I knew that my body energies were flowing freely and the negative effects of the chemicals inserted into my body through the chemo were being released.

I also took vitamins, garlic, calcium and aloe vera each morning. My life Purpose was devoted to healing my body so I could continue to serve others through my writing.

Some of the doctor's treatments were too uncomfortable. One was the use of a magnet placed on the lump. I did not continue it because I felt that energy was drained from my body. The acupuncturist accepted my choice.

Sometimes pressure from within on the lump would result from the treatment. I welcomed it because I knew the love pressure from the heart chakra was also in the treatment. Love heals!

My chiropractor was delighted with the results as I continued to visit him. At first I went twice a week and later only once a week. He was very supportive of my having surgery as recommended by my oncologist and surgeon. He said that getting rid of the insertion of chemicals in my body would bring forth greater health.

I found I had higher energy than many who go through the chemotherapy and as a result of the release of energy through acupuncture. I seemed to feel the results of the chemo less than others having treatment. Balancing the natural energy through these treatments was right for me.

The medical world has done wonders in the treatment of breast cancer. My personal opinion is that a mastectomy is too often performed because of the fear of the woman and the doctors' belief that to get rid of the problem for good is best. And that may be so in some cases. However, there is less and less emphasis on using that procedure. I determined I would not have one and the surgeon signed an agreement. The continued weaknesses and pain can debilitate the woman and take longer to overcome the experience. A positive attitude on the part of the oncologist, surgeon and chiropractor is most important. Women with this challenge are subject to great fear. The doctors can help alleviate that as they work with a positive attitude that the healing will occur.

I recommend that a woman find the doctor who feels like the right one to her. Be choosey. It is your life. Take care of it.

Thank God for medical knowledge that can help heal breast cancer.

Journal:

One day I shall rise in consciousness to knowing that all is God. I will leave behind thinking, feeling pain of body. But the truth for me at my level of consciousness now is that there is no one way that fits all people where they are now.

There are various ways depending on the soul's need. We each need a teacher, we need someone to understand how to clear the "stuff" so the Knowing from the Inner Self can be one's Guide eventually.

All is God. My body is pure Spirit. My thoughts are energized by that I AM. I find that truth often as I meditate, as I read spiritual books, as I study Goldsmith's philosophy and learn about the teachings of the religions of the world. But we are living in a human body and dealing with a world that requires use of our thoughts and feelings. To deny that world completely would bring neurosis or possibly psychosis. We live between two worlds. Our need is to balance the two to have a complete life.

Chapter IV

Spiritual Healing

As I faced my challenge and accepted that I needed to heal the separation between my daughters and me, I knew that spiritual healing by a practitioner of that art was needed. I had studied many spiritual healing methods, had practiced some through the years, had been convinced that to heal the body and mind the spiritual aspect of my life must be included. At this point in my consciousness expansion, I had been drawn to the teaching of Joel Goldsmith, founder of the Infinite Way. I had attended many classes, read and studied his books, and highly regarded the teacher of this philosophy whose classes I had attended. Her name is Elizabeth. I knew that she was very devoted to spiritual healing and thus would help me. So I called her early in my "adventure."

I realize that there are many methods being practiced now by spiritual and physical healers who are not always connected with the medical establishment. They are practicing various methods of energy healing such as Reiki, yoga, Tai Chi, etc. For some, meditation is not primary. For others, it is. Meditation was primary in Elizabeth's healing as well as studying and practicing the teaching of Goldsmith. Since meditation had been a primary practice of mine for 30 years and because I respected her highly and her interpretation of the Goldsmith teaching, I called her. What a gift she was and is!

I must add that as is usual with my spiritual journey, it is highly individualized. I go within to my Inner Spirit to get guidance for my choices and have found my own path. That path has included respect for the psychological aspect of any physical or emotional block I might encounter. The teaching of Goldsmith is not always interpreted as needing this emotional cleansing by psychological means. His is mainly a teaching for Mystics or for those aspiring to such a Path and much of this overcoming has already been done. I, on the other hand, had great respect for Carl Jung's psychology. Dream interpretation had been very helpful to me to explore my unconscious and get rid of many unconscious blocks. It was while I was in that "cleansing" process that I received my inspiration to write my first book. Therefore along with Goldsmith teaching I have combined the need to heal psychological blocks. My meditations with Elizabeth did exactly that as well as opening my conscious attempt to reach a level of relationship with my two daughters and healing any blockage I had to spiritual healing. And so Elizabeth's teaching and meditating individually with me was vital to my healing.

When I called Elizabeth and explained my challenge and my need, she immediately repeated what I had already heard and read but not fully practiced. She said: "Do not think about or picture the lump; keep meditating; read uplifting books; read the Bible; know that your body is God's body and that it has no destruction; don't share your concern with anyone, do not tell anyone.

"Keep your challenge a secret, as secret as possible. Fear that rises up in the hearer of the news can work as a deterrent to the healing," she added. She asked me to call her every day. And then she said, "Now we will go into meditation," and hung up.

I was experienced in meditation and so became quiet and immediately felt a deep vibration in my seventh chakra, a pressure. I knew our consciousness, hers and mine, were in deep contact. I stayed in that deep silence for an hour many times.

I called her each day for three weeks. After that it was every other day or so. She would teach me and then we would meditate in the Silence for various lengths of time. I was lifted up and felt I was healing physically, mentally, emotionally through the free movement of my Inner Spirit.

We discussed why breast cancer had almost become an obsessive fear among women even though more women die of heart disease than breast cancer. We agreed that the feminine was rising all over the planet and masculine dominance is being neutralized. Since heart and breast are so closely connected to the center of love, the Fourth chakra, we discussed whether this could be a warning to women to practice forgiveness of hurts by others, and let that love flow into mothering love for humankind. She knew of my reaching out to my daughters for a healing.

As we continued I realized I was at a crossroad of my spiritual Journey again. This was before I went to an oncologist. I wondered if I should depend on science for healing or on the Spirit, the Spirit of Love, within my consciousness. Or are both the same? Aren't they from the same source? Then I turned to an affirmation that quieted my concern and fear: "I see and feel God all around and through me. I let go of any fear. I let go of clinging to thoughts of the scientist. This body is God's body, not mine as a human. I belong to God—not to the physical world. It is my choice to trust God. It is the spark of God that I Am. 'Thou shall keep me in perfect peace whose mind is stayed on Thee.' I give up and let God be God."

I remembered momentarily that blessings and joy are mine. I declared: "I will be healed. God is all. I will have this healing. This growth is an illusion, an appearance that is not truth. I see it for what it is—a healing. This growth is an illusion, an appearance that is not truth. I see it for what it is—a negative to pull me away from the One. I let go and let God. I have need to fulfill my purpose. God is all."

It began to come through to conscious knowing that my spiritual consciousness was expanding as a result of my mental, emotional and physical challenges. Oh, not right away. It took several weeks of Elizabeth's teaching and our meditation and my study to bring me to this understanding. It took time. I needed to get some other things healed in my life to be totally healed. It took months of treatment, acupuncture, and many hours in meditation. And of course it all comes down to, "Love the Lord thy God and thy neighbor as thyself."

I wrote in my journal:

Love, not fear, is the answer. That is who I am, that is who we are. That is truth.

The following increased my Inner Awareness:

What an Awakening! Love, Love, Love! That is Who I AM. That is who everyone is. That is Truth. It will take me the rest of my life to be that Love, to live that Love at all times, in all situations. What a goal! It is in my giving love and receiving love that the healing occurs. Giving love to my small self from my Self. Feeling love from God. Giving love to everyone, every circumstance that I experience. My Path is Love.

For many Seekers referral to this Inner Spirit as God does not speak to them loudly as the use of Christ, Holy Spirit, kundalini, chi, etc. Because Goldsmith emphasizes the word God to cover all, it is often used in his writing. Those who have been students of and members of the Christian teaching find that turning to Jesus for healing is their Path. Well and good. Each needs his or her own language. For me the Christ is the Divine Energy, which is our life. Also Holy Spirit is the same as Christ Presence. All referrals to that God Presence needs a personal touch and may not be designated the same as another follower calls it. Each finds that word that describes this Divine Power within most helpful. We do have a choice. Because I was attending classes taught by Elizabeth and having meditation and private teaching, I used God as the Divine Presence mostly. Each has his or her own favorite word.

As I said, I was attending a class taught by Elizabeth. She often taught harmony as Truth. Not fear, not anger, no worry. Harmony is Truth. Discord is an illusion as well as imperfection. But neither has power. Perfection is God. She taught: "Be focused. The law of love, to love God first and neighbor and one's own self, is the healing Truth." A scripture came to me that illustrates this: "Do not be conformed to this world but be transformed by the renewal of your mind, that you may prove what is the will of God, what is good and acceptable and perfect." (Romans 12:2)[1] That I practiced to the best of my ability but I had a long way to go to perfection.

I read a book, *Sai Baba: The Embodiment of Love*, by Peggy Mason and Ron Laing. It says, "The cells of our body need love in order to be healthy. A distorted part of our body needs love just as a scraped knee on a child needs mother love to heal." How true, how very true!

Another teaching by Elizabeth: "Perfect balance is achieved when Spirit and thought are harmonized. Know that this experience you are going through "came to pass. Let it pass!"

As I went through my healing I often assured myself, "I am spirit, Christ is my teacher and my strength, I am also body and mind, which are instruments for God's Will in me."

It takes deep practice to drop all concern and keep one's thoughts on spiritual healing, on God's Love, on God as Truth, and to live the spiritual flow of Oneness in a world buffeted by egotism. Meditation at a deep level kept me centered most of the time. Consciousness of my Inner Spirit expanded.

One of my spiritual exercises was to visualize the Divine Energy moving up the spine to the crown chakra above the head. I did this as I breathed in deeply, held the Energy in place for a short time and let it go. This is Eastern, practiced by many Hindus and Buddhists and others. It always relaxed me.

Spiritual healing is as old as the human race although practiced in various ways. The Shaman illustrates this ancient knowledge. When our Spirit is blocked at a chakra, which symbolizes an important stage of our life, we may have discomfort, express negative emotions and be quite ill. I should like to refer you to Gary Zukav's recent publication, *The Heart of the Soul*. Coauthor is Linda Frances. In it they illustrate how our negative emotions may result in blockage of one of these Energy centers. Emotional awareness of the negative can transform a human life and blockages at these power centers need releasing. They and other authors are bringing this ancient truth forward to enhance the health of the seekers of spiritual, physical and emotional health. This Energy is God Energy and our life. (See *Sacred Contracts*, by Caroline Myss, also).

As an illustration, some years previous to my breast cancer challenge, I had a bleeding ulcer for three days before going to the emergency room at the hospital. There I had a Near Death Experience, which led me to a higher, deeper realm of Spirit and the loss of fear of death. The ulcer was at the location of the Third chakra, which is considered to be the last block to the full love power to be expressed in the Fourth chakra. I learned after research that a blocked Third chakra represents outrage over mistreatment by another. A loss of personal power is another interpretation. I had to heal what was blocking my Energy in order to move to unconditional love and compassion for all. When one is expanding consciousness, love needs to flow freely. Goldsmith teaches that disease will fade out of one's consciousness once hatred, fear or desire is released. Disease represents a belief of a self apart from God. An important teaching!

When our spiritual consciousness is blocked, then illness may occur. The healing comes as one knows "All is God" and one rests in faith and lets go of fear. This is not easy especially at the present time when reports of death from breast cancer are so rampant. The media can raise one's fear. I turned away from those dire predictions as much as I could.

Conscious awareness of our need to live in the Now—not the past or the future—is so important. When we move our thoughts from the past we let go of pain and fear many times. Of course there are happy and pleasant memories but we cannot always live on those. When we keep our thoughts on the future there is a certain amount of fear and anxiety. But when we live in the Now we are closer to who we really are, a spirit having a physical experience. Turning to the Now is turning in meditation to spiritual guidance. Healing will often come in body, mind and emotions. *The Power of Now*, by Eckhart Tolle, suggests that accepting the present moment is as one has chosen it. Work with it, not against it. The Now is your friend. How true that was for me as I was healing of my challenge.

It has been proven to me that finding a spiritual teacher who taught and meditated with me was so healing. I would suggest that if one is so guided they find a philosophy or a spiritual teaching that lifts one from fear, despair, anger, hate and asking "Why me?" If you are so led, pray and meditate often. If you have not learned to meditate this will be a good time to start. There are teachers and books that have this teaching. A retreat is another good way to learn to be silent. Accept Good as your inheritance. If one feels they have deep emotional problems to overcome, psychological help may be needed. As I have said, dream interpretation by a Jungian teacher was my choice. Jung's teaching was aimed at helping the seeker find the Inner Spirit or a religion that fit the need. Know that you are important to God's Purpose and to the world. Find your Purpose and go forth.

Another teaching from Elizabeth was that power was not in the cancer. Fear is not in the cancer. When one lives a spiritual, not a solely physical and mental life, one is relieved of worry. Life is eternal. The Spirit is in control. Surrender!

Sessions with her, meditation and her teaching, continued throughout the five to six months of my healing. In one of our sessions she taught: "Perfection already exists in the invisible, which is Reality. It is not physical healing you need so much as the raising of consciousness. As one's consciousness expands we are being made whole (holy). Our challenges are to raise our consciousness of Who we really are—the I AM. The dark is being filled with Light. Know all is well." Wow! That was not always easy. But what a teaching! A reminder to me to let go of fear and worry to enhance my healing.

The peace and love that expanded in my consciousness was a beautiful gift from this challenge. As Elizabeth taught me and meditated on the healing phase, I was blessed. I felt the power and joy of the Holy Spirit moving through me many times and my consciousness expanded. I pray that something in my experience will be valuable to other women who are facing this challenge.

I received a gift from this challenge. My consciousness was lifted to a higher, deeper level. To see the blessings that may accrue from the healing of a malignant tumor is a great gift. We can move to a depth of the I AM that we have not experienced before. And that conscious awareness will bring finer health physically, mentally and emotionally. We are then AT-ONE.

A mantra from Isaiah 61:1-3, repeated over and over, is healing:

The Spirit of the Lord God is upon me, because the Lord has anointed me to bring good tidings to the afflicted; he has sent me to bind up the brokenhearted, to proclaim liberty to the captives, and the opening of the prison to those who are bound. He has sent me to proclaim that the time has come when the Lord will save his people and defeat their enemies. He has sent me to comfort all who mourn, to give to those who mourn in Zion, joy and gladness instead of grief, a song of praise instead of sorrow. They will be like trees that the Lord himself has planted. They will all do what is right, and God will be praised for what he has done!

Journal:

I do not put my emphasis on healing the disease but on expanding consciousness of God. What happens to the disease will come as I center deeper and deeper. I let go of concern. Elizabeth emphasizes that this disease is not reality so I need not be concerned about it. God is unfolding the story of my life, and therefore it will be a happy ending as in a movie. Each morning I awaken with this mantra: "This is the day the Lord has made," and "Speak, God, for thy servant hears." I know that as my consciousness is my focus, is honored, all else will be taken care of.

Some Goldsmith teachings as interpreted by Elizabeth and understood by me:

Each one is the All-ness of God. Humility is needed in order to express that Allness fully. Surrender all that is apart from God. Blind faith is sweet surrender. Give up the mind as a power. Surrender! Get a clear signal from within—"Show me the way." Life need not involve suffering. Let go. Live in the Now. Do not borrow trouble for the future.

Wonderful teachings! I shall practice. All is well now. I have no pain. I am peaceful and quiet. NOW IS MY LIFE—NOT IN THE PAST OR THE FUTURE.

My sincere prayer for you, the healed and the searcher for healing, the healer and the "healee," is that your Journey will be filled with Light. Hold on to that wish. You have the healing Light within your consciousness, within your body, waiting to inspire you as well as the doctors who are working with your healing. No fear! Only Joy, Love and Divine expectations of a new Life.

Chapter V

Love Is the Answer

To write on love, a very ancient and forever popular topic, finds many seekers and finders who have searched for and found much written on it. They have lifted the consciousness of so many seekers. Our great teacher Jesus Christ gave us the ideal answer in Matthew 22:37-40:

A lawyer asked Jesus the question: Teacher, which in the law is the greatest? Jesus said to him: "You shall love the Lord your God with all your heart, and with all your soul, and with all your mind. This is the greatest and first commandment." And a second is like it: "You shall love your neighbor as yourself. On these two commandments hang all the law and the prophets."[1]

The interpretation of this scripture has bound together or divided many Christian groups. Each of us, whether we realize it or not, are seeking love from God, from our neighbors and indeed from our own small self as well as our Self. Our Self is indeed love but being in a physical body, living a life on this earth, has challenged that belief and practice many times.

One of the most human challenges is to love—not only one but many. There are those souls born into a human body who know Love from the beginning. Oh yes, we all do. But living our physical life with others who do not love themselves or do not know how to express love to another gives us our challenges. Peace, harmony, Spirit-centeredness is made more difficult as we live out our "four-score and ten." So most of us keep looking for It by various choices. For me, my choice later in life was to learn to love my Self and my neighbors (relatives, children, people in general) as my Self. That is a big challenge—to love others as we love God. Many times our love for God is watered down and we do not know how to love our neighbor.

Many of us, especially us women, are usually most drawn to loving our children through thick or thin. I thought that attachment to them and loving relationships with them was my divine expression of love at the deepest and highest. For some mothers this is true and the love is returned and the relationship is spiritually invigorating and satisfying. But for some mothers, a broken relationship will bring sorrow, pain but perhaps both mother and child grow in consciousness under that circumstance. It can either be the beginning of a healing or a freeing of the child to his/her own soul's choices. And that heals and releases the mother love to be devoted to others who are seeking it. After one's child reaches maturity, we release him or her to his/her own Purpose.

I learned so much about loving as I went through my challenge of breast cancer and after healing. So I would like to share some of my writing on this supreme topic of love and how my challenge affected my accepting love and giving love.

Our challenges in mental, physical or emotional health often opens the doors to great love and realizing that the closer we are to Oneness with that Holy Spirit, the God Presence, the deeper the love we have to share for our own self and for others.

Because my heart was open and my spiritual guidance was paramount during my healing, I shall quote directly from my Journal. I learned so much about love as I let go of disappointment over no response from one daughter and the response I received from the other one.

Before I start recording those insights I want to share what I have learned about relationships. I realized that every man and woman has suffered from broken relationships that were very important. And children, too. We have often assumed that loss through death is most painful. And it is for some. But to lose a relationship with children, parents, lover, spouse and others is equally if not more painful. Most of us try to revive the relationship but because each soul has its own Journey we may have to accept those broken relationships, from common blood sharing and from legal relationships. Those may not be as important as being who we really are. Relationships with our spiritual Purpose and expression of that may be more important this lifetime. I am always reminded of Jesus' teaching on this. (See Matthew 12:46-50) [2] He was fulfilling his Purpose and had to choose that first over his family.

As I record directly from my Journal I hope the deep feeling of love that was a part of my healing will touch the reader's heart. Each insight will be recorded in the order received.

Journal:

After a walk in the park next to my house and awakening, again, that God is Love, I received the following:

Love within does the work
Love within does the work
I of my own small self can do nothing
Love within does the work
It is love which I am
Love is who I am
Love is my Savior
I let go and let Love
I of my own self can do nothing
Love within does the work.

This is my mantra. I feel Love as I think, speak, recite this. Love is who I am and so is everyone. Love is near and dear. I am Love, Love, Love. I, God, is who I am. God is love. Love God. Love all. Love my small self. Love this challenge. Love, Love. If I speak with the voice of angels and do not have Love—it is worthless.

1 Corinthians 13: Love bears all things, believes all things, hopes all things, endures all things. So faith, hope, love abide, these three; but the greatest of these is love.[3]

Love God. Love God. Even though I walk through the valley of the shadow of death, I shall have no fear, for Love is with me. Love's rod and staff shall comfort me. Love protects me from fear, my cup overflows.

From 1 John I read and was uplifted:

"Beloved, let us love one another; for love is of God and he who loves is born of God and knows God." (4:7)[4]

"He who does not love does not know God, for God is love." (4:8)[5]

"No man has ever seen God; if we love another, God abides in us and his love is perfected in us." (4:12)[6]

"He who loves God should love his brother also." (4:21)[7]

"Greater love has no man than this, that a man lay down his life for his friends." (John 15:13)[8]

From my Journal:

As I turned to love and read scripture and other writings on love, it came to me that through the ages, because love has been misunderstood by much of the human race, it has been a puzzle. Now that I am awakening to love which I AM, I shall expand my consciousness. The Divine Energy within is love. But I do not always express it completely in thought, word or deed. My prejudices, my lack of giving to others, my need to be loved by others has kept me from this truth. Now I KNOW God is love. Christ is love. Jesus Christ gave great teachings on love. It is expressing it that is our task.

Love, love, love. Let it flow. I shall continue to let go of all social, religious and personal blocks to love. Love flows and I AM THAT.

Paul wrote:

"But speaking the truth in love, we must grow up in every way into the One who is the head—into our Christ Presence—from whom the whole body, joined and knit together by every ligament with which it is equipped as each part is working properly, promotes the body's growth in building itself up in love." (Ephesians 4:15,16)[9]

I shall study love not only from the Bible but from many books written to inspire me to love. One is *The Art of Loving* by Erich Fromm, and another is *Love, Medicine, and Miracles* by Dr. Bernie Siegel.

Two months after the last entry I was again turning to the past and not to the present, in the Now, and Love. It is an up-and-down Journey. I wrote:

It is interesting how easy it is for my thoughts to return to remembering past unhappy times in the middle of the night. When I could not let them go I arose and read spiritual material. I want to lose those memories of past negatives. However, as I overcome those memories I see them as bringing me a step closer to my freedom. Always the soul cries for freedom through love. In the past, as I met each challenge, I did the best I could given my lack of spiritual awareness. Oh, how I want to help others find their freedom in Spirit, which is Love. Love is the answer.

Another teaching for me:

My soul is speaking to me through this challenge. It is saying that blocking love has scarred my breast. I cannot function freely and clearly as long as I do not express the love which I AM. My soul is bringing me this realization over and over. I am removing the block to expressing love to all. Medicine will take away the physical appearance. Sharing my own awakening in love will help others who are going through a like challenge, I hope. I need to realize the need to feel and express God-given love is a healing.

I know that whatever the result of this challenge, it is another opportunity to expand my consciousness of love which I AM. Whatever the result, I shall be closer to my Source. That is what challenges are for. Our Soul's journey is why we are in a physical body. We choose to follow our Spirit's lead or refuse to. Each is free to choose.

When having a sleepless night I turned within several times but allowed concern for my health to interfere. Finally I repeated, "Let go, let God" over and over. I slept. That is letting go and letting Love Be.

Two old songs of love have been winging through my heart: "Beautiful Sunshine" and "Love Divine." Both old gospel hymns I grew up singing. These songs of love are love-centered. I am love, all is love. Love is the Kingdom of Heaven that Jesus taught is here and now. No wonder love is so misunderstood, misinterpreted. It can be quite frightening to dedicate one's life to love. And what is love? I am learning.

Last night when I was awake, I went into silent meditation. Each time divine bliss arose and filled my body. I am so filled with love this morning. When I awoke I could immediately go into the silence. I am learning so much about meditation for the treatment of cancer. I shall teach the benefit of meditation the rest of my life.

I was thinking on the big question—is cancer of the body a sign that love has been ignored, misused, misunderstood? Love heals. Through such a challenge, a gift if one realizes it, one may turn to looking at the lack of love, given or received, in one's own life and change to forgiveness and let the heart feel and send forth love to all. Unconditional love can be a lifetime task. Unconditional love is God Love. God loves all unconditionally. That is my task also.

I am convinced that the reason for coming to earth is to learn what love is, how to express, how to BE and how to Know. The two great laws that Jesus the Christ gave contain the greatest teaching on love. To fulfill those laws brings one to Oneness. But few of us can follow them one hundred percent of the time. They are: Love the Lord thy God with all your thought, mind and feeling, and your neighbor as yourself. That is a challenge that cannot be ignored.

Feeling love is being God-centered. Feeling and expressing love for everyone no matter what race, religion or choice of life style is our task. It takes a lifetime to come to that level for most of us. It is not just loving the outer, loving one's church teaching, loving one's family, loving one's country. Well and good if carried out from the heart, but "mind-love" will not fill one's longing to know love. I know that I need to practice love for the rest of my life no matter what the circumstance. It is a deep subject. Each must answer his or her own questions about love.

In reading the book The Art of Loving, I am reminded that this body is love. If by thought, word or action I leave out love, the body reacts in disturbance, maybe disease, sickness or mental aberration. Love is who I AM in Spirit and body. Love flows through the Prana, the kundalini, the Divine Energy, which is the life and love of my body. Opening to that Divine Energy brings us more love—from others and to others. That is why we come to birth, to learn to live in love. Then our life will be complete. All the hitches we experience are outside the field of love. Many of us choose experiences not motivated by love and unhappiness is experienced, for our basic Self—Love—protests. The true mystic lives from love and not from thought. The love of God is an intense feeling experience of Oneness.

The following excerpts from my Journal were written after I had surgery and was declared healed by the surgeon:

Loving kindness is the pearl of great price resting on one's heart. Trust love only. Throw away all other keys. Love the Lord your God with all strength, thought, spirit and heart. This is the key to all doors in the Father/Mother's house. This is the Ark of the Covenant. (The Ark of the Covenant was a precious box in which the Jew's covenant with God, received by Moses, was kept. It was the center of the benevolent presence of God to his people.) Thus, one's heart is the Ark of the Covenant of Love.

Love is all there is. Love is life, truth and joy. Oh, how long it takes us humans to learn that. We find our love in other people. We believe that to love another human is the epitome of love expressed and received, but it often plays out for we expect the other one to be God-like. And that expectation often fails. We look for love from animals, our children, our leaders in religion and government. And they, many times, fail to fulfill our hunger. When we finally "get it," that the love we seek is within, is our Holy Spirit, then we can detach from expectations from all others. We can have love, be love and appreciate whatever another person can give. We can express it without any preconceived expectations.

Love is life. Love is all. Love is from God and to love God first will change our loving of others as well as our selves. That love will be my guide for earth experiences as well as in higher dimensions.

I have gone through a crucifixion. Many who do not realize that a resurrection of love felt, known, expressed to one's self as well as to others and the world can be the result of a crucifixion. Love elevates the consciousness of the world.

I shall nurture the truth of love being All. We are surrounded by Light Beings, Angels, who are helping open us to this consciousness.

Allow love to stretch the computer of your heart. The Tree of Life is the eternal reality of love. Devotion births the process of love. Observe the peace and power that is at work within consciousness. Be a witness of God's love. Follow your heart. Follow your dream.

These love messages are the guiding principles I try to follow to the best of my ability and they are never ending for love is eternal and being in a physical body makes expression of love so important to our health and our "ongoingness" of our spiritual path. Love for our self is so primary and as we get rid of our blockages we feel it more freely and give it to others. God is love. Think "love" when you think of God. Read scripture using Love instead of the word God. That will open your feeling of love and enhance your Journey.

Just a last note or repetition on the Divine Energy, Holy Spirit, kundalini. All are the same. All are the love that is our life. It is love that heals, that lifts our consciousness to serving others, that brings us the high bliss that we experience when that Energy is unobstructed and flows freely up our spine through our chakras. Meditation, devotion to our spiritual path, and baptism by another spiritual human centered in God can bring it alive and change our life. But with that must be a change of thinking. It must include love, for that Spirit is Love in its fullest degree. Bliss, Enlightenment, Mystic Marriage will result and our life will be complete, at least this time around.

"If I speak in the tongues of mortals and of angels, but do not have love, I am a noisy gong or a clanging cymbal. And if I have prophetic powers, and understand all mysteries and all knowledge, and if I have all faith, so as to remove mountains, but do not have love, I am nothing. Love is patient; love is kind; love is not envious or boastful or arrogant or rude. It does not insist on its own way…it bears all things, believes all things, hopes all things, endures all things…and now faith, hope and love abide, these three; and the greatest of these is love. (1 Corinthians 13:1-7,13)[10]

CHAPTER VI

Healing Through Forgiveness

If you truly love yourself and others who are equally subject to making mistakes, forgiveness is automatic. But most of us who reach out or in for the Spiritual Journey are older and have already accumulated a few experiences from and to others that have affected us negatively. Or we have not asked for forgiveness from those we have harmed, many times, unintentionally or through our ignorance of what this life is all about. When we realize that true forgiveness is a part of our Journey and let go in love for ourselves and/or another, we have cleared our consciousness for an expanded Journey of love.

As I was about 81 years old when I had this challenge there were a "few" people who I needed to forgive. But first I knew forgiveness of myself was in order. I had been on a conscious spiritual Path for 31 years. I had meditated many hours. I had studied Eastern and Western religions and had written 12 books and had published 6. Most were written from a symbolic understanding of scripture. I had taught many seminars based on my books and I felt that I was following that Inner Guidance. But there was much more. Expansion of consciousness never ends.

My challenges in relationships had largely been centered on my ex-husband and my daughters. I was always seeking peace but complete forgiveness was still waiting. I knew my daughters had forgiven me of many mistakes. Now I felt I had to go through this physical challenge to awaken me to my need to ask their forgiveness and reach a peaceful relationship with them. My ex-husband had already passed on and I had forgiven him and asked for his forgiveness years previous.

I also needed to forgive our government and its sending my son to Vietnam to serve a useless cause and giving up his physical body. I needed to forgive the ignorance of the war consciousness of our leaders and our citizenry.

Over the years my daughter Carolyn had been very unhappy with me and had separated from contact for maybe several years. Sue was closer but in time had cancelled our relationship. Now I faced the challenge of cancer and needed to forgive and ask for forgiveness.

I was aware that I had lived from a mother complex that needed healing. I had tried to gain their forgiveness before but had not freed them. This I needed to do.

I learned that separation from family, old friends, religious friends may result when one steps on the mystic path. But as I have written, I was not ready to give up on my daughters. So I wrote them deep heart searching letters, asking for forgiveness and telling them of my challenge. I expressed my love and asked them to forgive me.

From my Journal:

I wonder, is the greatest lesson we humans learn in earth living based on relationships, loving one, lack of, broken, and with the Divine? I mean, relationships with other humans as well as with our own Self? How many of us try to satisfy our longing for that divine relationship with our Creator, with God, by our relationships with people? Yes, that seems to satisfy for a period but a vacant feeling may remain. Sometimes it seems that we are happy, but the rela-

tionship usually comes up wanting—never satisfying our inner longing.

When we find our Self, our Holy Spirit within, it makes all the difference in our intimate relationships. With love of our Inner Self, our love for others takes on a different hue and forgiveness unblocks any separation.

I have told the results of my reaching out to my daughters in the chapter on "Healing Physical and Emotional Pain." I learned so much about love and forgiveness that I count those experiences as primary in my spiritual Journey. Teachings from a hurt heart are our deepest and finest lessons. And often take us to Oneness of no separation from other people and primarily from God. This separation brought me to peace as I dealt with forgiveness of each one and of myself. The mother complex was healed. My daughters have chosen to act from the expression of their own soul's guidance.

During this time I was studying Caroline Myss' book *Anatomy of the Spirit* with a friend. The chapter on love including teaching on forgiveness was just what I needed. I wrote the following as we studied that chapter:

Forgiveness is mending any thought, word or feeling that has been expressed which separates the Christ Light in one person or group of persons from another. We are all One—what I AM is the I AM of everyone. When we are separated from each other by holding a grudge or anger or hurt feelings, we are more disturbed than the person we do not forgive.

My forgiving was put on hold for many years for my husband. Until I realized that it was separating me from my Inner Self, I kept remembering his actions and words. Then I realized that I was separated from my Holy Spirit by keeping those memories active. I began to see him as doing what he thought was best. I knew that I needed to forgive him and my self. My non-forgiveness was hurting me the most.

To forgive is Divine, for to totally forgive is to totally love my neighbor as myself. If I am One with God, I cannot be unforgiving, for God is love. And with love paramount in my life, forgiveness comes naturally. Peace of heart, body and mind come with forgiveness.

I have been forgiven many times by others. I ask for forgiveness when I realize I have offended. But sometimes I may not be aware of my offense. The trick is to remain in love all the time but being human that is next to impossible.

I thank God for forgiveness from others but primarily from God for I am separated from that love when I hurt another or do not forgive.

Forgiveness is to allow the love that I AM to understand another's actions and words as coming from some deep need in them, or deep hurt, that is being released through personal problems and their lack of self-confidence or lack of sensitivity to the needs of others. Loving the other and forgiving are the only genuine ways to clear the path between us.

Sometimes one must speak or write to the one from whom forgiveness is needed. A genuine note, written in love, to ask forgiveness is accepted and forgiveness comes forth from that one. We are all One. When I do not forgive another I have not forgiven myself and am affected first. I also give them freedom to forgive me. God forgives as we forgive and the slate is clean. We are forgiven!

In The Lord's Prayer, we read and recite: 'And forgive us our debts as we also have forgiven our debtors.' That means that our debts are separation from realization of our Inner Spirit. This refers to spiritual forgiveness, not thought forgiveness or action. If we realize our Inner Spirit presence, we forgive others readily for they have that Inner Spirit also, albeit they may be unconscious of It.

This line from the Lord's Prayer became truth for me. I had many debts. I needed forgiveness from God and God guided me to forgive myself as well as others in my life. I was clearing my consciousness of blocks to love, which needed clearing so the heart chakra could function and rise and heal the lump that was damaging my health. Breast cancer may be related to lack of forgiveness of self and others as well as not loving the Lord our God and our neighbor as ourself. Hindering the flow of love from one's heart chakra brings challenges to one's physical body. The fourth chakra, love, needs unblocking.

I shall now give some ideas for forgiving that I have taken from recently published books. I have quoted Caroline Myss and others on forgiveness. Forgiveness liberates the psyche and soul from the need to "pay back." This releases the feeling of being a victim. Forgiveness can heal and indeed may bring a miracle.

From Roger Walsh's book, *Essential Spirituality*, we find several deep teachings on forgiveness. Again forgiveness of self for offending another is most important. Forgiving our small self heals. When we understand and accept our part in another's offense we freely forgive both our self and the one we have offended. My need to forgive myself and my daughters was needed in thought, word and deed.

I also recommend Bernie Siegel's *Love, Medicine & Miracles.* A short quote (page 197): "You have to remember that you cannot change anyone. You can only change yourself. When we speak our forgiveness to another the whole relationship can be healed. Unconditional love heals."

Suffering can be the open doorway to transformation as soon as we can forgive ourselves and others. We are well on the way to psychological, physical and spiritual healing. Love shines through!

Our need to be forgiven by others is really based on our need for God's forgiveness. Scripture quoted from Jesus' teaching is so valuable. Our praying to God to forgive our trespasses is basic to our peace of mind and as we pray to be forgiven and to forgive we are strengthened. God forgives as we love and seek forgiveness from others.

A few scriptures from Jesus' teaching strengthened me.

Matthew 6:14,15: "For if you forgive others their trespasses, your heavenly Father will also forgive you; but if you do not forgive others, neither will your Father forgive your trespasses."[1]

When Peter asked Jesus how often he should forgive an offender, Jesus replied: "Not seven times but, I tell you, seventy-seven times." (Matthew 18:21)[2]

Mark 11:25 teaches when we pray we should forgive. If we hold anything against another we should forgive as God forgives us.

And it is recorded in Luke 23:34 that Jesus asked God to forgive those who were crucifying him. For, he said, they know not what they do. We too are crucified, buried in a dark cave, but forgiveness frees us to ascend to our spiritual goal. Let go of the pain of crucifixion by another and send love and forgiveness. That is the mystic's journey.

Let love flow from heart to body and be healed both physically and spiritually. And life will open to one's Purpose, which is to love God, one's small self, and one's neighbor likewise.

Chapter VII

Dream Time Related to Healing

Many years before this challenge came to me I had been guided by my dreams to new writing assignments, to solving of problems, to guidance of how to react to a situation. A Jungian master interpreter had helped me interpret my dreams on a regular basis for several years. From that I had let go of blocks to my conscious realization of who I AM and I was inspired to start writing books. The inspiration to write my first book, a metaphorical interpretation of the Book of Revelation in the Bible, came to me as I meditated. This happened after I had several years of cleaning out my subconscious with dream interpretation. My purpose was revealed to me. Since then I have taken my dreams very seriously and have learned how many guide me, support me, inspire me. I am very adept at covering up unconscious truth. My dreams sneak in while I am asleep and I remember, interpret and follow my inner Guidance. Some, of course, are more difficult to understand and may not reveal a teaching so far as I am able to decipher the meaning.

This is an introduction to the part that my dreams played in opening me to what was blocking my love, which I believe was at the base of the reason for the breast cancer. At the beginning of my conscious realization that the lump was serious I began seeking what in my personal relationships might be blocking love. And, of course, the lack of peaceful loving relationships with my daughters surfaced. Relationships needed healing. As I listened and followed the teaching from my dreams I was rewarded. This was part of the healing treatment I gave myself.

The first dream came through soon after I recognized my need to seek a professional decision about the lump I had found on my breast.

Dream:

> I was visiting in a home. The wife was not a part of her husband's fundamentalist religious belief. He was dressed in suit and tie and was going to church. She was not going.

Interpretation:

I am still carrying the absolutist belief that my masculine side is uppermost. My feminine side does not agree with it. I shall bless it and let it go, the masculine choice. I shall rest on the feminine aspect of my consciousness and reach out for help. The man reminds me of my former husband whom I have forgiven and released.

The analysis made me realize that I had been ignoring the lump and the need to start healing it because my masculine side had been in control. I was fine, I would think, I can heal it through spiritual means. My feminine side of needing to seek help was revealed in this dream.

* * *

Before I started dealing with the lump I had been writing a book entitled *A Mystical Journey Through the Psalms*. This next dream came soon after the first one.

Dream:

> I was traveling with a group of people and visiting a family. The oldest woman remarked that I was not as

present during the visit as in the past. That bothered me and inferred that I was not as loving as usual. I walked through a large building to the entrance where the car was parked to continue on my trip with the others. I heard the car start when I came to the street. The group was loaded up and driving away. A trailer contained two women sitting and a young man standing. I yelled but only the young man looked back and waved. They did not come back for me. I was left alone. My baggage went with them.

Interpretation:

I am being prepared to be alone. This symbolized my three children leaving me. This was showing me the loneliness of my life. My consciousness was reminding me of my aloneness and the need to deal with it. It opened me to a conversation called Active Imagination by Jung. I would ask a question of my inner Being and get an answer.

Active Imagination:

I asked if I should let go of my daughters completely. My son had already left his physical body. My answer: You are still holding onto some grief in losing them. Let go and let God. Find peace within. Let go of any guilt. All is in the divine plan. Forgive yourself and them. You are holding onto something that needs releasing.

Later I realized: I love my Self and my daughters enough to forgive them and my small self. That will heal the wounds of the past as well as this wound in my breast. I forgive my self and them. From pain in relationships has come my deepest spiritual teaching and expansion. In Self-love is the healing of this knot. And Self-love is based on unconditional love for others. Self-pity and separation from loving others has brought this challenge. I shall contact my daughters and repair those relationships.

After this I turned to feelings of deep love and thoughts for my daughters. I realized the lump on the breast and this dream had revealed my next step—seeking mending of the separation. A clearer spiritual Path was opening. I could not shut down this love I had for them. It must flow in order to heal them as well as fulfill my physical and emotional need. Soon I would write or call each as I found their addresses and/or telephone numbers.

On September 12, my 81st birthday, I had the following dream:

> I was giving a lecture on kundalini energy to a large group in a lecture hall. The people were scattered around. Some came in late. I explained the process of raising the Spirit within which will bring a high level of spiritual knowing. I felt perfectly comfortable in speaking.

Interpretation:

Since this came the morning of my birth date, is it telling me that this is why I was born—to bring this teaching to a diverse group? Did I come to life in a physical body to reveal this deep secret to Western Christians? The Bible is the text and the deep teaching is there. The secret of the kundalini, love, is basic to life. My newest published book is being read by those who have not known about the effect of raising this energy as part of one's spiritual journey.

This dream added to my decisions to seek a doctor and start the process of healing by medical means. My Purpose needed a healthy body. This began the journey, the long road, of examination, chemotherapy and surgery. And more importantly healing physically, mentally, spiritually and emotionally. I also contacted each daughter, told of my challenge, asked for forgiveness and sent love to both.

Accepting my responsibility for seeking peace between my daughters and myself and acting on it began to release me from that blockage. I went into medical treatment as well as deep spiritual meditation with my Teacher. And my dreams changed.

Before starting the chemotherapy, I went through a Dark Night of the Soul. I let worry block my close touch with my Divine Being. Not for long, though. I awoke later on that night with full consciousness of my Spirit.

These dreams came as I slept and healed. There were two:

> At a meeting of several people who were discussing spiritual matters, a tall man entered. His name was Cosmo. He entered into the conversation with deep knowledge. I supported him in his remarks. When the meeting was finished, he came and asked me to meet him for a drink. I accepted.

Interpretation:

Cosmo is short for Cosmos, which means order and harmony. This dream is saying that I have much in common with order and harmony. My Christ is order and harmony. I need to eat and drink with That, which is my future as well as the Now. I commit my small self to order and harmony. No fear, just relaxation, commitment and support. Since I often have a young man who cares for me come to me in my dreams, I see Cosmo as a divine messenger, perhaps Jesus Christ. I have teaching to do and am cared for.

I was reassured that I was on the right Path and had Sacred Guidance.

Dream:

> I was on a street in a busy city preparing to give a talk. The organizer gave me a sign to begin. I had loud speaker equipment and started speaking about God. Several people stopped to listen. I was explaining that God is Mother/Father—both female and male. And then I said,

> "Actually God is neither. God is It. We have made God one or the other in order to understand, but God is neither." I felt honored to be teaching the passers-by in order to help them on their spiritual way. When I awoke I was uplifted.

Interpretation:

My task is to spread the word publicly to all who pass by, who will listen. I have the Word, the Christ, within as all do and this dream gives me the "go ahead" sign to speak out. This teaching of moving God from the masculine category to a balance of the masculine/feminine, and then to the neuter "It" is the progress of the message I am to deliver. I am in my rightful place. This is support for my writing and for my speaking to help others on the Path.

This dream reaffirmed my Purpose—to teach the passers-by from a higher, deeper level. This reassured me that I was back on my spiritual path and would speak and write in the future—I had a future, I would be healed.

Dream:

> A short dream about going into the mountains to attend a meeting. When I arrived, Hillary Clinton saw me and came to me. I told her I would wait to be seated when my friends arrived. She nodded and went to a table and brought a candy bar to me. I thanked her.

Interpretation:

This dream brought me a feeling of love and attention from a loving woman. The feminine is taking care of me. It gave me peace, love and assurance that I was where I was meant to be. I still had much to learn and express, but I would be taken care of. I was getting psychologically prepared to have my first chemo. A certain amount of fear and worry was disturbing me. This dream reassured me that all was well.

* * *

As I went into the chemo treatment my sleep was disturbed by physical and mental disquiet. I thought after two chemos that the lump would vanish. I was not at peace, however. I had no dreams worth recording after this one (November 8) until December 28. The following dream was meant to relieve me of my sorrow over my daughter Sue not responding to my reaching out to her. This dream depicts us as being together.

Dream:

> Sue and I were riding in a car into a high school parking lot. I was driving. There was broken glass in the driveway, which I swerved to avoid but ran over some. We discussed why there was so much broken glass in the parking lot.

Interpretation:

Sue and I were traveling together on our spiritual journey. We are in an immature place at the time. We are meeting some blocks on our Journey. The broken relationship cannot be avoided completely, but our souls are traveling in the same direction. We are in an immature (high school) phase. We will graduate from it. Sue is in her rightful place and so am I.

This dream helped me accept, with love, Sue's freedom to not respond to my letters. I accepted that she had her own life and we were traveling together on the level of immaturity, of high school learning. The broken glass interfered with our Journey. Broken glass blocks the clear journey but we can avoid it by forgiveness and loving.

A month later I had three dreams in one night that gave me deep instruction. I was back on track. The blocks to my realization of who I am were revealed. It is unusual to remember more than one or two dreams in one night that had unsettling endings!

Dream:

One dream was in a shopping area, another was in a cluttered house, which I was cleaning up and where I was propositioned by a preacher, another was in a wilderness area where I was looking for beauty of nature but forgot to pay the price and therefore did not find it. All of these dreams lacked light and beauty of Spirit. I realized I had been awakened to a truth I had ignored.

Interpretation:

Materialism (shopping), cleaning up my house (consciousness), not being interrupted by religion (preacher), and not appreciating nature enough (not paying the price) are all very human experiences. These are recognized in my past and I hope I have let go. Any dream that carries a negative connotation should be examined and then forgotten. That is a cleansing of the unconscious.

The three dreams indicated that I would have disappointments when focusing on the ways of the world. Commercialism, sex and money or lack of it, is the way of the world. Cleaning one room indicated that my consciousness would be cleaned up by my own efforts. Finding myself in the mall and disappointment in not experiencing the beauty of nature (God) indicated a potential separation from my Journey. I let go of the carnal mind (belief in my small self, ego) and return to the business of God's plan for me, my purpose. God spoke to me through these dreams.

* * *

As with most women who have chemotherapy, I lost my hair. I have always been proud of my brown curly hair as one of my strongest beauty characteristics. So I grieved some. A dream assured me that all was well.

Dream:

My hair has grown back. It was dark brown and long. I was surprised and delighted.

Interpretation:

Recovery is assured again. Hair is a symbol of Spirit flowing from the seventh chakra. Hair symbolizes vital force. Symbolically a shaven head indicates loss of sexual desire. Women's hair symbolizes the feminine authority. I am assured I have that by the grace of God.

* * *

I had received four chemotherapies and the surgeon had declared the lump was smaller and surgery would be the next step. I wrote, "Prayer, meditation, spiritual healing, acupuncture, chemo and surgery—the full treatment. I am healed." This was written on February 18. Surgery date was March 4. An involved dream assured me of a safe journey home.

Dream:

I was in Mexico walking through a jungle to get to the border to return home. A man and a woman went ahead and a woman friend followed. It was night and very dark but I had a light, which I used sometimes. The leading couple turned off the path and we came to a river. They walked through the river of Light. The man came back to help my friend and me through. We arrived at the border. The couple found some food and disappeared. We had to wait but finally were served. We were waiting to board an airplane to fly home when I awoke.

Interpretation:

I have been in a foreign, dark place. I must walk through a primitive forest, follow the masculine and feminine, have no fear of the river of Light, and know that the oncologist (male) and surgeon (female) will lead me to the cross-over to Home.

Eventually the two doctors will disappear and I shall be ready to go Home and pick up my normal life. The prediction that I would "fly" home was wonderful.

A dream that pictured me as very vulnerable came to me:

> I was walking alone through a snowy passage to China. A young man came to help me. The land strip I was walking on ended at a building, which was my destination. I came to a pond of water. I did not want to walk through it. I saw footprints around the edge leading to the door of the building, which was China. I started to go that way. Awoke.

Interpretation:

The young man is the acupuncturist who is helping me cover my vulnerability. The snowy path I had to walk to get to the building that was in China was reached safely. I am being assured that the China connection to acupuncture will cover my vulnerability to exposure.

Acupuncture, which is from Chinese medical practice, was healing me also. My choice to have acupuncture to release my Divine Energy throughout my body led me to the entry door for my passage. A reassurance that acupuncture was most important in my healing came forth.

* * *

March 4, my date with surgery, was set. On March 4 my Journal was:

> *This is the day the Lord has made. Let us rejoice and be glad in it.*

And I Knew It. I had been silently assured the day before that three Light Beings would be in attendance at the operation to direct and lead the surgeon and attendants when needed. I wrote:

This is God's body sent to do God's work and as long as my Spirit needs me to express in this physical body, I shall be here in it.

The night before surgery this dream came:

A friend and I went to a gathering in an auditorium. We could not find two seats together so we separated. Later, one opened up near her and I moved. Two young men spoke but several women were chattering behind me and I could not hear. Then Deepak Chopra was on stage for a brief time. He then came and found a seat behind us. When the program was over, I thanked him for the teachings in his books. He thanked me humbly and then said he was going to lunch.

Interpretation:

I am in a large company of women who are not paying attention to the speakers. This dream tells me that I am healed. Deepak Chopra is the "healer's healer" for this time. He symbolizes healing. I am being assured that the healing Spirit is with me. My friend is love, which is the healing agent also. This predicted: All Is Well!

* * *

The operation was successful. Only a few lymph nodes were removed and had no sign of cancer cells. It took me a while to recover but my friends and loved ones supported me. I gained strength and was healed in more ways than one. Emotionally my one daughter Carolyn was with me and in close touch by telephone. Her loving attention was so needed. Sue had been released to her own divine journey, in love and understanding. I was ready to branch out into a new life.

On March 16, I dreamed of taking a trip to Hawaii, which reassured me that all was well. I only needed Oneness to "fly."

Dream:

I was traveling in Hawaii with just one "dressy" dress. When I was at the airport ready to return home, I showed a picture of myself to the clerk. She remarked that I look more and more like my mother. I was surprised and asked if she knew her. She said, "Yes."

Interpretation:

My mother symbolically is God-Light that I reflect. Hawaii symbolizes beauty, ancient religion, fire of the volcanoes where the goddess Pele resides. All symbolic. My Path has been with the vital force called Mana in Hawaii; kundalini, chi in the East. It is Light, which surrounds the body. I need only one such body to be dressed well. I am returning Home. The Light of the Presence, my Light body, is all that I need in which to be dressed for the beautiful earth experience represented by Hawaii.

A very important dream followed on April 16. I can still recall a faint memory of awakening to it.

Dream:

I was traveling with a young girl. We spent the night in a hotel. Next morning I went out to do an errand leaving the young girl to get ready to travel. When I returned, she was in a state of confusion, had unpacked and was repacking. I helped her and tried to get her ready. A man came in who had rented the room and was to occupy it after we left. He was calm and organized. The room, I was told, was mine to use as I desired.

Interpretation:

This dream could have several interpretations. Since I was in contact with my granddaughter, who was going through a confused time, it could have referred to her. Or it could refer to my confusion in my own physical and mental consciousness (room). I am not organized enough to continue my journey. The young girl was a quality in my thoughts and body that prevented me continuing on my journey. The young man would then be the Christ figure that is often near to help me in my dreams. Either interpretation brings me bread for my Odyssey. The young, confused girl may be revealing some childlike characteristic that needs maturing in my self.

I still have not completed my journey. My immature level of consciousness may bring confusion but the Christ Spirit will be there to befriend me as It enters my consciousness. These divine messages from the Christ, the young man, Jesus Christ's teaching supported me many times.

On the first of May after my healing I traveled to Cleveland from Denver to present a seminar on my book, *The Bible and Kundalini Energy*. The three-hour presentation in the afternoon brought out many questions addressed to me. I often answered "I do not know. You will find your own spiritual answers if you center and listen."

While at home I had more calls from women seeking answers to their spiritual and physical needs. I knew that my writing would be enriched as I finished the book on the Psalms. Reflections from my challenges were contained in it.

Dream:

> I was traveling with two women and two children. I was driving. The car needed repairing so I took it to a garage. They loaned me a pickup truck to drive. I took the friends to a store and let them off and went to park the truck. I joined them at the store. Later I went to get the truck where I had parked it. Could not find. Looked and looked up one street and down another. Finally, I went back to the store. The owner suggested I call the police. They said they had towed it away because it had no owner. I got directions of how to find the police parking lot. We were starting to walk there when I awoke.

Interpretation:

Traveling is symbolic of my spiritual journey. When I borrow a vehicle for it, I lose my conveyance. I cannot find it for it is not mine. Taking care of others who travel with me will bring confusion and loss on my journey if I feel too responsible for their safety. "Let go to the owner of All—God The Good" is the message. I of my own self can only release those seekers to the Holy Spirit of each one who is in need. Each will learn his/her own lessons and go on to greater awareness. When one reaches out to me for healing, I shall release all to God and know their need is met. This is being Love.

After a similar confused dream I again realized that I had allowed the negative experiences of friends and relatives to impinge on the soft peace of my soul. I thought: "I love each one and release them to God's love and peace. I have done my part."

My last recorded dream deals with the Mystical Marriage. The coming together of one's masculine and feminine nature in Oneness of the Spirit is a Mystical Marriage. If this is unfamiliar to you, the following explanation of Mystical Marriage taken from Evelyn Underhill's book, *Mysticism*, explains it well:

Mysticism is the perfect consummation of the love of God. It is the art of establishing one's conscious relation with the Absolute. It is the soul's surrender to the embrace of perfect Love. It is the soul's unity with All That Is. There is no longer a soul/God relationship but only God. To remain in that high estate may be for a moment or for days. It depends on the seeker's guidance. The mystic comes into that relationship inadvertently sometimes. Having that experience is never forgotten.

Now to my dream. A beautiful close to a chapter of my life that opened me more fully to that Divine Oneness to which my Spiritual Journey has led.

Dream:

I had met a young man and was attracted to him. He asked me for a date and I accepted. He was to come to my house. To get ready I went upstairs to my very pleasant room. It was large with bed, chairs, a round table with family pictures on it. I started getting dressed for the date. I chose a beautiful slip, found the right dress, fixed my hair and face. I was taking my time. I knew I wouldn't be ready on time. I saw him drive into the driveway. I felt deep love for him. I was not ready to greet him. I finished dressing. As I finished, he and my family were coming up the stairway. When he entered the room, he saw the pictures on the table, examined them, and asked questions about them. I explained who they were. We finally left. We were walking down the sidewalk toward the light area, arm in arm. I asked him about a restaurant. I loved him and knew he loved me. I wondered if we would marry. Awoke.

Interpretation:

As I am reading this dream two days later, I am feeling love bubbling up. It has come to me that my feminine is in love with my masculine, my Godhead, and we are almost One, almost married. Going arm in arm toward the Light is going toward unity in the Light. Being completely in the Light is the Mystical Marriage. That is a Divine level and I am almost there. My large room upstairs indicates a high, expanded consciousness. He came up to find me. The pictures were the spiritual family with whom I have lived in order to grow spiritually. His patience with my lateness reflects God's patience with me. This young man, the Christ, came to claim me. He has been my guide and my beacon in dreams as well as in waking life. The slowness in dressing showed my reluctance to take the final step of the Mystical Marriage. But he and I were going arm in arm toward the Light. We were One.

This dream showed that I am healed and on my way to Enlightenment, living in the Light, being at One with masculine and feminine Energies. I have not completely become One but am walking toward the Light.

I am firmly assured that direction from my dreams was very important for my healing journey. Overcoming the challenge of blocking love has healed me and taught me spiritual awareness of Who I Am. I have greater Love, Light and Oneness.

Challenges are for our own benefit to lift us to a higher spiritual level if we are desiring that. Our total self—both unconscious, conscious and super conscious—are involved. The lessons we need to learn as to what blocks to let go of are revealed step by step on our spiritual Journey.

We are all on a spiritual Journey consciously or unconsciously. Dreams from our unconscious are important in that Journey. Listen, interpret, and learn your directions. There are many teachers willing to help you through classes, books, retreats, dream interpretation counseling. Find your Way!

HOPE

We have known
Sorrow and Pain of
Mind.
But hope springs
Eternal
When Spirit we
Find.

CHAPTER VIII

Active Imagination as a Healer

Active Imagination is a new term for many so I shall give a definition I have gleaned from the study of A.I. and by practicing it.

A Jungian analyst taught me Active Imagination developed by Carl Jung. Jung equated the unconscious with the One Mind. Active Imagination is entered into consciously in an effort to engage the unconscious in dialogue with the ego. It is a receptive attitude toward the unconscious. One asks a question, becomes quiet, listens for an answer from the unconscious. Writing the question and answer was my method. Other methods may be to paint, draw, speak into a recorder. Creativity can be accessed in this manner. However, if the ego is too strong, a valid answer may not be received. Not until one has found that One Mind, the Christ within, the Holy Spirit, and one does not ask but waits for guidance, is the help infallible. I shall show how this affected my Journey through healing breast cancer.

Active Imagination was an important element of my healing. I had practiced it assiduously ever since I had several years of dream interpretation by a Jungian analyst. Many times when I went for an appointment he would ask to hear my "actives" before hearing my dreams. They were very important for the opening of my unconscious to the talent of writing books, which developed while I was seeing him. Active Imagination opens up the channel from our conscious mind to our unconscious and the more unblocked the unconscious the clearer will be the answers to one's questions.

The process is connected with one's ability to stop the thoughts in deep meditation and go into the silence. Many Seekers need lengthy practice of meditation so the thoughts are quieted and one can "hear" what the answer is to the question posed. The Spirit speaks and One's consciousness hears and records accurately. Many of my spiritual directions and guidance have come from this Inner listening.

Because this may be a new healing method for the reader, I should like to present some teachings from a book written by my Jungian dream analyst, Jeffrey Raff. The following is taken from his book, *Jung and the Alchemical Imagination.*

"Jung was a great student of Alchemy. He taught his clients this art of Active Imagination and believed deeply in its effectiveness. A.I. (Active Imagination) is divine imagination. It guides one to living a moral life, to devoting oneself to service to others, to receive revelation from one's Holy Spirit.

"One definition of A.I. is 'The name of an Internal Talk of one person with another that is invisible.' It is really communion with one's Self.

"Usually the participant is on a quest. A quest for insight into one's needs through Inner Wisdom. It is imagination and consciousness of Spirit combined. A uniting of the masculine (intellect) and the feminine (intuition) to bring forth the Self, which guides one to a higher purpose."

I remember that it was during these sessions on dream and active imagination teaching that I received guidance to write my first book, an interpretation of the Book of Revelation, in 1980. I had been a student of symbolic interpretation of the Bible and a deep meditator for 12 years. As I wrote that book

I depended on this Inner Voice many times to give me an explanation of the scripture. I realized that my creative ability from dream interpretation and practicing A.I. brought forth my creative work. It was a successful book when published.

Dr. Raff writes, "Disease, being spiritual in its origins, has the power to create images, and therefore can only be treated successfully in the realm of the imagination." (Page 75)

He adds that Active Imagination remains a potent force in the treatment of disease. Disease, he writes, is never a purely physical event, but includes the spirit also. Healing needs the spirit, which is contacted in the A.I. process. He quotes Dr. Arnold Mindell, a Jungian analyst, who wrote the book, *Dreambody*, which says that the physical and spiritual are important in healing.

My experience with A.I. sometimes brought an image, sometimes a feeling, sometimes a physical sensation from within but more generally it brought a message to write from inspiration, to write what I "heard." A.I. can inspire art, ideas for healing, music composition, scientific truths, creativity of all kinds. And can accrue from paying attention to one's Inner Guide. It is reported that many inventors brought forth advanced spiritual truth as well as scientific inventions from silencing the thoughts and listening and recording.

Lastly, healing of the negative archetypes one has allowed to control one's life can result. Vital truth about which of our archetypes are positive and which need healing can come through the A.I. Caroline Myss goes into great detail about archetypes in her book, *Sacred Contracts*. She was also a student of Carl Jung's teachings.

Now let us go to examples of my A.I. experiences that affected my physical as well as spiritual healing. Early on as I dealt with what I needed to do in order to find peace, I turned to an Inner inquiry, an A.I.

I asked:

Should I let go of my daughters?

Answer:

You are still holding onto some grief. Let go and Let God. Find peace within. Let go of any guilt. All is in divine plan. Forgive yourself and them.

Question:

How?

Answer:

Change your thinking. Free your love to be active. Be aware of your feelings toward them and forgive. Turn to Me and listen. Release any negative emotions.

I then asked if the separation was the will of God.

Answer:

Divine teaching is coming forth. Good is coming to them and to you through this separation. Be in God's will. If you are to be together it will be God's Will. They need this time to find their own Paths.

Because at this point I was trying to find the reason for the knot in my breast and if it was related to my withholding forgiveness and love from them, I asked that question.

The answer was "Yes."

I accepted that the blocking of love for them had been conducive to the growth of the tumor on my breast. I realized that this challenge came to me to expand my consciousness of loving all and to serve through the writing of books from this deep spiritual perspective. I accepted then that as a mother I had given the best I had to give but it was not perfect. But now, even though having lacked perfection in my mothering, I was free to go forward in love through forgiveness of my self and them. I decided to get in touch with both and ask for forgiveness.

Later I again asked:

Dear God, what do you want me to do for Thy daughters?

Answer:

Love them, forgive them, release them and contact them.

I then wrote a letter to Carolyn and thanked her for the love she had expressed in a birthday card. I asked for forgiveness of my neglect and expressed my forgiveness to her. I then waited to get an address for Sue, which came very soon.

In the same month I let fear surface over the examinations for cancer. I was guided to Let Go. And then I asked:

Why was I chosen to have this challenge?

Answer:

You chose—you chose—not to teach others primarily but to teach you. You will be able to teach others through this experience. Healing will come. Let go!

After it was determined that I should have chemotherapy I was instructed by a nurse on the hazards and negative results. I was confused and asked why I had this confusing experience.

Answer:

I AM in the medicine, I AM the chemo, I AM the discoverer of its healing effect, I AM the effect, I AM the healing. Nothing is separate from Me. Go forth. There is no separation between medical and spiritual healing. Those who are healed by the medical world are my servants. They need to give their attention to Me and their Journey in order to avoid disease striking again. Each soul will be born again until it is free to express the Truth in word, emotion and deed. I AM all.

I recognized that there is no complete healing without Spirit recognition.

It was now December 1. I had accepted this need in September. I was having chemo every three weeks. My meditations with Elizabeth continued and acupuncture was begun. I was impatient though. I asked:

> Dear God, that which I AM, why is my body not healed immediately?

Answer:

> Your teaching goes on as you heal. You are healed but your acceptance of that is not clear. You still cling to the medical decision and are tinged by the society's fear of cancer. Consciousness of your Inner Being has expanded, though. Let that become Truth, is your need.

I asked:

> How can I do that more completely?

Answer:

> Let go of human belief that the flesh is separate from the Spirit. When you fully accept that your flesh is Spirit, healing will be complete.

I then asked if I should quit going to doctors.

Answer:

> Not yet. That time will come. You are healed spiritually.

Question:

> The evidence is that I am not healed. The lump is still here.

Answer:

> You keep it there with your attention to it and touching it. Your confidence in the medical world is enhanced as it gets smaller. You do not need that evidence. The flesh is God manifest.

Again I realized that my body is spirit and blocking the acceptance of that Truth had brought this glitch. Both the physical and the spiritual must be cared for. A balance is needed.

Around December 25, I am always touched by deep messages as I turn within for guidance. Inspiration to write my first book came at this time of year.

An important message came forth:

> Love is Spirit, but human beings find love a mystery and sometimes put it on the back burner to simmer until it is needed to bring peace and joy to a dying world in their experience. Love is that all-pervading consciousness which is God manifest. Continue on your path.

The first of a new year brought forth a question to my Inner Guide as why I needed further medical treatment since the Spirit had declared me healed. Again I was told I needed the full human experience in order to teach others by a complete description of my experience. I was reminded:

> God is health. God has no illness.

I knew that my choices to not follow the scripture in Matthew 22:37-40 had made this challenge possible: Love the Lord thy God with all your heart, soul, mind and your neighbor as yourself. This had not been always fulfilled. I believe that Love was what I had not practiced in the situations with my daughters. It was learning to really love that this challenge had taught me. It would seem I was a slow learner. The human scene got in my way. But I was healed.

I was surprised, as I reviewed my Journal, how many times a deep truth had to surface before I accepted it completely. To be open to these divine messages and to make them truth for my Odyssey became my aim. As my consciousness expanded, these truths came to me with more strength. My Path required my accepting and experiencing these truths.

At times I became very bored with the whole process. My energy was often low from the chemicals in the chemo treatment. As I found myself in a depressive state I heard from within:

> All is well. Take care of your own life. All others will be taken care of. BE at One. No separation. Be and Be and Be. Let Go. No responsibilities. Just Be. Let come what will. Know all is well. You are healed. Your work goes on. Be! Be! Be!

Then I realized again that I had backslid. I repeated: I Am. The Lord my God is my Holy Spirit. I AM that. I then asked My Self what I lacked to find this Inner peace.

Answer:

> Your physical condition, race consciousness, lack of personal separation from all that is not God. Turn within for longer periods of meditation. Do that often. When you don't, worry can take over.

I realized then that indeed my long periods of meditation with Elizabeth had been reduced. I decided to spend more time in private meditation.

Since I had not heard from my daughter Sue in spite of my sending her many letters, I recognized my pain from her lack of response. I turned within in A.I. to hear this:

> You need to let go of any expectation that Sue will respond to your letters and your expression of love. She is not free to respond. But do not let go of her. Continue to send love, healing and prayers for her happiness, but know it is your Spirit, not your emotional, physical needs that are reaching out. See her as a Child of God and bless her as you would anyone who comes to mind. She is your spiritual daughter now. Bless her. Let go of

> personal expectations. Have loving interest in her welfare but free her. Face the truth that she cannot reply to you. Love her and let her go.

This message finally convinced me. I quit expecting any answer from her and freed her to the power of the Spirit that lies within her. She is her own Self.

After the operation and being declared healed by my surgeon, I rejoiced and thanked my Holy Spirit for all the messages, the answers to my uncertainty as I went through the healing. It was now two weeks after the operation and I had a message from my Inner Self that was very important. I shall nurture the truth of love being All. We are all surrounded by Light Beings who are helping us through our crises if we are open to them and do not cover them up. Our Inner Being gives us Truth for our Journey.

I received:

> Allow love to stretch the computer of your heart. The Tree of Life is the eternal reality of love. Devotion births the process of love. Observe the peace and power that is at work within consciousness. Be a witness of God's love. Follow your heart. Follow your dream working within consciousness. Be a witness of God's love. Follow your heart.

All of these messages led me higher and higher, deeper and deeper! I shall continue to meditate on peace for my daughters. Both are living their own spiritual Journey. All that is peace and love will be expressed by them in their life experiences.

My life pretty well settled down to routine after the successful operation. I was writing the Journal account of my breast cancer experience. I had given a Seminar in a church in Ohio. I was healed! I had attended a conference on healing, medicine, spirit and science. I was relaxed. But there are always challenges to help us expand our consciousness. I had periods of sleeplessness.

I went within and asked:

Dear Mother/Father, teach me about the wakefulness.

Answer:

Let it go. Flow with it. Do your work. Read, write, relax, let go. Flow with it. Accept it as a gift. A parenthesis in Eternity. No problem. Flow. Accept. Don't fight. This is your life. Get up and read or write during these periods. Meditate. Listen, Center. God speaks. Follow this routine. Listen. It is part of your life. Accept.

And then I realized again:

A change of routine comes with expanding consciousness. You are not the same consciousness as you were eight and a half months ago when this challenge started. You are changed, thus your physical, emotional and mental life is changed. Look for the differences and be thrilled.

That was a beautiful message from my Inner Self teaching and guiding me.

On July 4, four months after the complete healing, this came forth:

FREEDOM, FREEDOM, FREEDOM. Freedom from fear! Freedom to love! Freedom to follow the path that my Spirit has designed for me. Freedom! We are free, free, free. It takes spiritual centeredness to know that. I am free! Thank you loving friends, loving angels, loving Beings of Light. Love! That is Who I AM. Thank you, thank you.

All is Well, very, very Well!

Psalm 46:10,11

"Be still, and know that I am God!
I am exalted among the nations,
I am exalted in the earth.
The Lord of hosts is with us;
The God of Jacob is our refuge. Selah."[1]

Chapter IX

The Healing Power of Creativity

I had never considered my self as creative for I always attached that term to artists, musicians, inventors, writers who had brought something new to the world. And I had done none of those. I rested on intellect, I thought, for my choices and guidance and I was successful—as the world turns. Oh yes, during my first years of focus on finding my spiritual Path I would write short paragraphs answering a question that I later learned was Active Imagination. But that was not creative, I thought. After I started my spiritual choices beautiful teaching through poetry started coming to me—all spiritual teaching—and I recorded it. A surprising gift and one that raised my consciousness higher and higher. I didn't recognize at first where it came from—thought it was intellectual. And then I knew I was being taught spiritual truth for my own expansion of consciousness first and for others as I shared it. My intuition, my Sixth chakra, was open and spirit and intellect had combined to bring it forth. I was delighted.

It was several years before I found my talent, or Spirit revealed my talent, to write spiritual books. I recognized that it was a talent long dormant and as my books became popular I recognized my life's Purpose—to write and publish metaphorical interpretations of the Bible.

That changed my life. Everything moved into place—retirement, travel, study, financial support, inspiration and deeper meditations on who I AM. My life took on a new aura. Oh yes, I still had human problems to heal but my Inner Self was giving me blessings. I was fulfilling my Divine Purpose.

I had lived a full life. I had had my ups and downs. I had learned so much from my human experiences through the years, which gave me a rich inner knowing of the human condition. I was 63 years old when I started writing books. As a result my interpretations of Biblical scripture touched the needs and the hearts of thousands of readers.

Oh yes, so much of my inspiration came not from my intellect but from my sixth chakra—the wisdom chakra. This chakra at the influence of the pineal and pituitary glands in the crown and in the forehead has been named the creative chakra by East and West spiritually inspired seekers.

The results of bringing together one's Inner Spirit consciousness and one's thoughts is health producing as well as depression lifting. Physical healing as well as mental peace. God is creator and I AM God is our mantra. The Voice within inspires us. I was inspired to write my first book by that Inner Voice.

Creativity, when accepted as spiritual essence, gives birth to the mystic consciousness and when we reach that divine goal our true Self comes forth in expression, our true Purpose for our soul's taking on a physical body is revealed. And to serve others is basic to our living in a physical body. Creativity is a moral virtue even though it may not be accepted as such. Many confuse creativity as a purely intellectual process. If it arises from thought power only, it is not the creativity I am describing.

It is suggested by many truly creative artists—for we are all artists—that the Spirit is the Creator. We are only the device used by Spirit. Creativity causes one to lose his/her small self and find the Inner Self as primary. When we realize that everyone is capable of being creative by expressing the Self through body, mind and soul, one is well on the way to being a true Mystic. If one allows fear to surface, that Inner Self is lost and true creativity flies out the window. Rest in that Inner Spirit and let your creativity speak. Be Guided.

During my six and a half months session with healing breast cancer I also was healed emotionally, spiritually and mentally. As I have recorded previously this healing advanced my consciousness to a deeper level and my creativity thrived. I had started writing a book entitled, *A Mystical Journey Through the Psalms*. As I felt strong enough I continued to write and finished the book soon after the final healing through the operation. And that creativity was part of my healing process. My doctor agreed.

Let us go now to a few entries in my Journal that indicate the blessings I had from creativity.

As I studied Psalm 119—this was before I had accepted a need for medical examination—I made a list of the steps that were needed for my Infinite Journey. I wrote:

> *I am studying Psalm 119, preparing to interpret it for the new book. From it, I received a list of steps that are needed for my Infinite Journey. Some of them are: A need for peace in a difficult situation; see the Presence in others; meditate; handle negative experiences with faith and Knowing; discover blocks in personality; let go of thought of person, place or thing that separates me from my Path; be guided from within; serve others; let go of all fear.*

I am sure that following that list to the best of my ability affected my healing.

As I have indicated elsewhere I was having dream interpretation by a Jungian professional and Active Imagination were my messages from within as I had written my first book many years ago.

After I learned through medical exam that I had a cancer on my breast I decided to continue to write on the book as I learned more spiritual Truth. Also writing would take my mind off of any fear and anxiety I might experience. I wrote:

This creativity adds to my peace of mind, for when I am being creative I am listening and writing from my Inner Center. I wrote a chapter on Peace this morning, which helped me in my present challenge.

As I wrote I would receive deep messages meant only for me at first. When I wrote a chapter on "Finding Your Purpose" and I used Psalms to teach it, I realized again how I had been blessed in finding my Purpose for taking on this physical body.

At the same time I was being taught by a teacher of Goldsmith philosophy. As she taught me I was reminded that in interpreting Psalms I had found the steps to Enlightenment: Believing, Faith, Knowing, Being. These are steps that many go through in seeking Enlightenment. I had followed them. During this crisis I was into Knowing and many times Being. This writing had reminded me of who I am and how I need to expand spiritually.

One of the chapters was entitled "A Prayer for Old Age." I used Psalm 71 as that message. Verse 9 expresses the fear of many older people, including my self, in depression. Verse 9: "Don't throw me away now that I am old, nor desert me now that my strength is failing."[1]

I wrote:

Fear of abandonment, fear of illness, fear of death. Those fears can be alleviated by a deep experience of the Spirit.

Yes, that strengthened me.

On December 27, I wrote:

When I am not feeling well, I often become well by being creative. I was feeling dizzy yesterday morning. I had break-

fast, went to my creation room, read a little, and then meditated. I then remembered, "Creativity heals." So I started editing, putting my thoughts on improving what I had written and was healed. I had not written for a week or two and needed that deep centeredness to feel better. God pouring through me brings balance.

I finished the last chapter on the Psalm book entitled, *The Mystical Marriage*, and put it away to be typed in final form. I had been inspired to write a book some time previous, on the Sermon on the Mount, a special teaching by Jesus as recorded in Matthew 5-7. I began studying various books I had and reached inspiration to begin. This was after the operation.

As I studied the Sermon, I was inspired by Matthew: "Blessed are the peacemakers for they shall be called children of God."

I wrote:

I interpreted peacemaker as referring to the individual being at peace within themselves through meditation and prayer and coming to Oneness with God. One touch with the Presence can bring "conversion" or "born again" in a spiritual way. True peace between people and within oneself comes from forgiving. To bring peace—silent thought of the All-Power of Love and Wisdom—will cause trouble to melt away. This influence of the Word spoken silently will bring peace.

On March 23, I wrote:

I am beginning to feel the anticipation of starting on the new book. I shall wait, listen and write when Guided. A repetition of the realization of guidance is often necessary for me. A slow learner! The right time is coming forth.

On April 28, I wrote that the new manuscript *A Mystical Journey Through the Psalms* had been typed in final form and I was very proud of it. It is interpreted in light of one's Mystical Journey and I am on that Path.

On July Fourth, I wrote:

> *Freedom, freedom, freedom. A day of rejoicing in the mountains attending a spiritual retreat. Freedom from fear! Freedom to love! Freedom to follow the path that my Spirit has designed for me! Freedom! We are free, free, free. But it takes spiritual centeredness to know that. I am free! Thank loving friends, loving angels, loving Beings of Light and Love! That is WHO I AM. Thank you, thank you!*

All is well, very, very Well.

And I was so "blest" as I continued on my creative Journey. I am still on It as I am inspired. I finished the Sermon on the Mount book in several months and continue to write. Thank you, God, for Creativity.

CHAPTER X

Spiritual Realizations

This chapter, the final one, will contain a list of the deep learnings I have accepted that came to me so that I could continue my Journey to Enlightenment. I wrote:

> *The shift from total centeredness on the healing and to my spiritual growth is a detachment and a new beginning. I find myself wanting to share my good news and at the same time accepting that this challenge is in the past and the future is in the Will of God. Healing and centeredness will continue but on a different level.*

A review of my learning from the experience seemed in order. I wrote:

> *This review of my Odyssey may not describe the journey for everyone faced with this challenge but perhaps it will give some guidance to those women facing a like challenge.*

The healing of the physical, emotional, mental and spiritual disturbance recorded in my Journal included:

- A broader, deeper experience in meditation and prayer.
- Turning in love as the answer to the healing need.
- Reading books on healing of disease through love, which reinforced my own belief.

- Keeping a positive attitude that I would be healed, that I was already healed. Positive thoughts and feelings were experienced several times a day.
- Daily contact at the beginning with a spiritual teacher and meditations with her.
- A weekly class to study spiritual teachings of Joel Goldsmith.
- Spiritual prayers and treatments by friends through love for me.
- Medical treatment—chemotherapy and surgery.
- Alternative healing through acupuncture, chi gong, laser, healing touch.
- Accepting the deep teaching this challenge had for me.
- Keeping a Journal to share with other women with a like challenge in a book I would write.
- Opening to Universal Spirit completely for guidance in major decisions.
- Being creative in continuing to write a new book, *A Mystical Journey Through the Psalms*.
- Experiences of Oneness with God, neighbor and my Self.
- Development of an expanded Purpose—to teach others that Love is the healing Energy.
- Accepting and Knowing that Being at One is All That Is.

Books I studied:

The Art of Loving, by Erich Fromm
The Path to Love, by Deepak Chopra
The Practice of Spiritual Healing, by Joel Goldsmith
Love, Medicine and Miracles, by Bernie Siegel
Joy's Way, by Brugh Joy
Anatomy of the Spirit, by Caroline Myss
The Bible
The Celestine Vision, by James Redfield
The Return of the Dove, by Diadra

This is not a total list but the ones that inspired me during this challenge. And all is well!

All those who are facing a crisis in their life may find help in the inspiration and the books I have listed. Listen! And find your healing Path!

ADDENDUM

A personal message to the readers of *A Spiritual and Medical Odyssey*:

The recalling of my Odyssey through the ups and downs, the doubts and fears, the ignorance and the learning, the joys and bliss has been a great gift to me and I hope to you the reader. This Odyssey is recorded in humility for it is God's message spoken, as near as I was able to receive and express, through my consciousness and through my pen.

My sincere prayer for you, the healed and the searcher for healing, the healer and the healee, is that your Odyssey will be filled with Light as mine has been. And do not immediately discount that wish. You have that healing Light within your consciousness waiting to inspire you as well as the doctors who are working with you. Let fear go! Know that whatever your future, it is divinely preordained.

This is my last insight on the subject of healing breast cancer, and other forms also, through the grace and love that you are. Be that and continue your own Odyssey into the Light. Thus, one comes to the beginning of a new life for oneself as well as for those one touches.

I wrote in my Journal:

> *The human condition is one that the soul incarnates into for various reasons or purposes. Each has a unique purpose. The mystery for each soul is Why? Why? Why? And some are never enlightened, recognizing the Light within. It is a tedious journey for many. For others, it seems to be fairly simple. All are in God's Way for each is God. The God Presence is Who you are and that God Presence sees you through*

the "valley of the shadow of death" when your spiritual Purpose may awaken.

By the grace of God, we can arise, we can resurrect with greater wisdom and realize Who We Are. Then our real Path begins.

The wisdom of the ages is slow in coming to many of us. We go through many deep "valleys" until one day we awaken and really live or we leave the physical world and have, by the grace of God, another chance through reincarnation to overcome the shadows and find the Pure Light which we are.

Disease, so-called tragedy, loss of loving relationships, loss of fortune, loss of health, loss of knowing who we are, may come to each of us. All may be described as tragedies, but the loss of ego due to spiritual healing of the small self is a lovely loss. Yes, oh yes. For when we recognize that loss, we have awakened. God is waiting in the wings for our turnaround. We have these various challenges in order to awaken to the truth of our existence. Through God's grace we find our Path and follow our Inner Guide, which brings us the joy, love, plentiful rewards of our physical/spiritual life. All is planned for us. Our part is to open to the plan and follow. Then the Light shows forth and we recognize It. And joy and love reign supreme.

"You shall love the Lord, your God, with all your heart, and with all your soul, and with all your mind, and with all your strength," and "You shall love your neighbor as yourself. There is no other commandment greater than these. (Mark 12:30,31)[1]

LOVE IS THE ANSWER.

St. John of the Cross wrote in *Living Flames of Love*, "Love wounds, love heals, love transforms one to the Highest Peak of Oneness, of Bliss."

And so It Is!

MAY THE LORD JESUS CHRIST, THE BUDDHA, ALLAH, AND ALL THAT IS BE WITH YOU FOREVER!

Glossary of Terms

Chakras – Center or whirls of energy at certain locations in the ethereal (energy or auric) body or spirit body, located at endocrine glands.

Christ – The spark of Divinity within each consciousness. The Inner Voice; the Counselor, Prince of Peace. Jesus called It the Father.

Collective Unconscious – The totality of beliefs, thoughts, memories, feelings and experiences of the human race.

Consciousness – An awareness, a knowing of the Divine, the Christ, of God. Conscious awareness of God, of the Spirit.

"I" – The spiritual Presence within individual consciousness.

Kundalini – An Eastern word for divine energy. The fire of regeneration located at the base of the spine. Called Chi, Ki, Life Force, Holy Spirit by other religions.

Meditation – A stopping of the thoughts by focusing on one thought, one thing, on the breath, on a mantra. A touching of the inner Divinity in the Silence.

Mystic – One who centers his/her life on knowledge and activity of the Spirit. The mystic follows the invisible presence that lies within and that forms the other experiences.

Race Consciousness – The beliefs, actions, mores of that society in which one lives that affect one's choices.

Regeneration – Uniting body, mind, spirit into Oneness with God.

Self (capital "S") – The Inner Divine Presence, the Spirit, the Christ.

self (small "s") – The ego; the human self; belief in self-will.

Bible Verses

Chapter I	1. 1 Corinthians 12:9
	2. Philippians 4:13
Chapter II	None
Chapter III	None
Chapter IV	1. Isaiah 61:1-3
Chapter V	1. Matthew 22:37-40
	2. Matthew 12:46-50
	3. 1 Corinthians 13
	4. 1 John 4:7
	5. 1 John 4:8
	6. 1 John 4:12
	7. 1 John 4:21
	8. John 15:13
	9. Ephesians 4:15,16
	10. 1 Corinthians 13:1-7,13
Chapter VI	1. Matthew 6:14,15
	2. Matthew 18:21
	3. Mark 11:25
Chapter VII	None
Chapter VIII	1. Psalm 46:10,11
Chapter IX	1. Psalm 71:9
Chapter X	None
Addendum	1. Mark 12:30,31

Bibliography

Chopra, Deepak, *The Path to Love*. New York: Three Rivers Press, 1997.

Diadra, *The Return of the Dove*. Dallas: Wings of the Spirit Foundation, 1995.

Dossey, Larry, M.D., *Recovering the Soul*. New York: Bantam Books, 1989.

Elder, Dorothy, M.A., *From Metaphysical to Mystical*. Denver: Doriel Publishing, 1993.

Elder, Dorothy, M.A., *Revelation for a New Age, the Book of Revelation*. Marina del Rey, Calif.: DeVorss & Co., 1981.

Elder, Dorothy, M.A., *Song of Songs and Enlightenment*. Marina del Rey, Calif.: DeVorss & Co., 1988.

Elder, Dorothy, M.A., *The Bible and Kundalini Energy*. Denver: Doriel Publishing, 1997.

Elder, Dorothy, M.A., *Women of the Bible Speak to Women of Today*. Marina del Rey, Calif.: DeVorss & Co., 1986.

Elder, Dorothy, M.A., *Born Free, Reincarnation and Karma*. Denver: Doriel Publishing, 2000.

Fromm, Erich, *The Art of Loving*. New York: Harper and Rowe, 1956.

Goldsmith, Joel, *Awakening to Mystical Consciousness*. Lakewood, Colo.: I-Level-Acropolis Books, 1998.

Goldsmith, Joel, *Living Between Two Worlds*. New York: Harper and Rowe, 1974.

Goldsmith, Joel, *Realization of Oneness (The Practice of Spiritual Healing)*. New York: Carol Publishing, 1995.

Greaves, Helen, *Testimony of Light*. Essex, England: C.W. Daniel Co., Ltd. 1996.

Jampolsky, Gerald, *Love is Letting Go of Fear*. Berkeley, Calif.: Celestial Arts, 1979.

Joy, Brugh, *Joy's Way*. New York, J.P. Tarcher, Inc., 1979.

Jung, Carl, *Psychology and Religion*. New York: Bollingen Foundation, 1969.

Krishna, Gopi, *Living with Kundalini*. Boston: Shambhala, 1993.

Love, Susan, M.D., *Dr. Susan Love's Breast Book*. New York: Addison-Wesley, 1995.

Mason, Peggy and Laing, Ron, *Sai Baba: The Embodiment of Love*. The Hollies, Wellow, Bath, England: Gateway Books, 1993.

Myers, Tona Pearce, *The Soul of Creativity*. Novato, Calif.: New World Library, 1999.

Mindell, Arnold, *Dreambody*. Boston: Sigo Press, 1982.

Myss, Caroline, Ph.D., *Anatomy of the Spirit*. New York, HarperCollins, 1996.

Myss, Caroline, Ph.D., *Sacred Contracts*. New York: Harmony Books, 2001.

Myss, Caroline, Ph.D., and Shealy, Norman, M.D., *The Creation of Health*, Three Rivers Press, 1993.

Ornish, Dean, M.D., *Love and Survival*. New York: HarperCollins, 1998.

Raff, Jeffrey, *Jung and the Alchemical Imagination*. York Beach, Maine: Nicolas-Hays, Inc., 2000.

Redfield, James, *Celestine Prophecy*. Hoover, Alabama: Satori Publishing, 1993.

Siegel, Bernie, M.D., *Love, Medicine and Miracles*. New York, Harper and Rowe, 1990.

St. John of the Cross, *Dark Night of the Soul* (Translated by E. Allison Peers). Garden City, NY: Image Books, 1959.

St. John of the Cross, *Living Flame of Love* (Translated by E. Allison Peers). Garden City, NY: Image Books, 1962.

Underhill, Evelyn, *Mysticism*. Cleveland: World Publishing Press, 1957.

Walsh, Roger, *Essential Spirituality*. New York: John Wiley & Sons., Inc., 1999.

Wilber, Ken, *Grace and Grit, Spirituality and Healing*. Boston: Shambhala, 1993.

Yogananda, Paramahansa, *Autobiography of a Yogi*. Los Angeles: Self-Realization Fellowship, 1969.

Zukav, Gary and Frances, Linda, *The Heart of the Soul*. New York: Simon & Shuster Source, 2001.

TAPES (AUDIO)

Chopra, Deepak, *The Path to Love*. New York: Random House, Audio Publishing, 1997 (two audiotapes).

Hoffman, Janalea, *Mind-Body Rhythm, Music for Healing*. Unity Village, Missouri: Unity School of Christianity, 1996.

Moran, Michael, *Prepare to be Healed, Meditations for Before and After Medical Treatments*. Unity Village, Missouri: Unity School of Christianity, 1996.

Siegel, Bernie, M.D., *Healing Images* (Narration by Bernie Siegel, music by Jerry Florence). Santa Monica, Calif.: Hay House, Digital Stereo, 1990.

Woodard, Kevin; chiropractor, *Acupuncture: A Billion People Can't Be Wrong*. Lakewood, Colo. (Call 303-989-5740.)

BIOGRAPHICAL SKETCH

Dorothy Elder has been a student of world religions, the metaphysical and mystical path of many Seekers, and has combined Christian teachings and those world religions in many of her books. The teachings of Carl Jung, her personal experiences with the Divine Energy, and her expression of creativity have all added to her own personal spiritual journey. Dorothy has experienced marriage and children and a career as a counselor in public education. She is the author of fourteen books. Her Purpose is to share spiritual insights with those who are led to seek their own Path. Her experience with the healing of cancer has given a new dimension to her life and to her writing. Dorothy has published seven books, many of which are based on an esoteric interpretation of Scripture. Revealing aspects of her own personal spiritual Journey has given inspiration to many others.

Other Books by Dorothy Elder

Revelation For A New Age (The Book of Revelation)

Women of the Bible Speak to Women of Today

From Metaphysical to Mystical

The Song of Songs and Enlightenment

Proof of the Truth, The Spiritual Journey of Grace Faus

The Bible and Kundalini Energy

Born Free: Reincarnation and Karma Examined Again

ORDER FORM

Please send __________ copy(ies) of *Healing Breast Cancer: A Spiritual and Medical Odyssey* to:

Name ____

Address ______________________________________

City ____________________ State _____ Zip __________

Phone ____

The price is $12.95 plus $2.00 for postage per book.

Mail to: Doriel Publishing Co.
Dorothy Elder
2557 S. Dover #75
Denver, CO 80227